Atlas of Flexible Bronchoscopy

I would like to dedicate this book to my family for all their support and encouragement despite the endless evenings and weekends spent on this book. A special thanks to my wife, Mala who created some of the initial anatomical drawing for this book.

Atlas of Flexible Bronchoscopy

Pallav Shah MD FRCP

Consultant Physician and Honorary Senior Lecturer
Royal Brompton Hospital, Chelsea and Westminster
Hospital and Imperial College London, UK

CRC Press
Taylor & Francis Group
Boca Raton London New York

CRC Press is an imprint of the
Taylor & Francis Group, an **informa** business

CRC Press
Taylor & Francis Group
6000 Broken Sound Parkway NW, Suite 300
Boca Raton, FL 33487-2742

First issued in paperback 2022

First issued hardback 2019

© 2011 by Taylor & Francis Group, LLC
CRC Press is an imprint of Taylor & Francis Group, an Informa business

No claim to original U.S. Government works

ISBN 13: 978-1-03-247758-9 (pbk)
ISBN 13: 978-0-340-96832-1 (hbk)

DOI: 10.1201/b13458

Visit the Taylor & Francis Web site at
http://www.taylorandfrancis.com

and the CRC Press Web site at
http://www.crcpress.com

Contents

Preface

'Striving for excellence in the care of our patients'.

My ambition for this book is to provide a simple step wise approach to flexible bronchoscopy. I have linked gross anatomy with the radiology and correlated it to the bronchoscopic findings and view. This approach should assist the bronchoscopist with both diagnostic and therapeutic procedures. Safe practice is also of paramount importance and is a key theme throughout this book.

Introduction

Bronchoscopy has become an essential tool for the respiratory physician. The original fibreoptic bronchoscopes were primarily utilized for visualizing the airways and also for sampling. The modern video bronchoscopes provide high-definition images of the airways so that even subtle lesions are recognized. The procedure has also expanded from simple diagnostic procedures to therapeutic procedures. The development has seen the therapeutic capabilities progress from palliative treatment of endobronchial tumours to asthma and emphysema.

Equipment

The bronchoscope is essentially a flexible tube consisting of fibreoptic bundles, channels for instruments and a number of wires for manipulating the distal end. The bundles of optical fibres carry light to the distal end in order to illuminate the airways, and further bundles transmit the image back to the eyepiece (Fig. 1.1). The modern video bronchoscopes have a charge-coupled device (CCD) chip at the distal end which captures the image and is subsequently transmitted to the monitor (Figs 1.2–1.4). The resolution of the image is excellent and continues to improve, with some scopes providing very high-definition images with digital magnification options. There are also hybrid devices for special circumstances, which use the fibreoptic bundle to transmit the image back towards the head of the bronchoscope. In this case, the CCD is located at the head of the bronchoscope, which then transmits the image to the monitor. The hybrid setup allows the space of the chip at the distal end to be utilized for

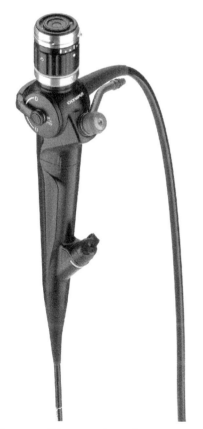

Fig. 1.1 *Fibreoptic bronchoscope with eyepiece.*

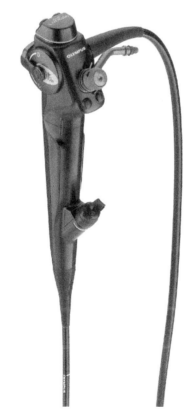

Fig. 1.2 *Video bronchoscope.*

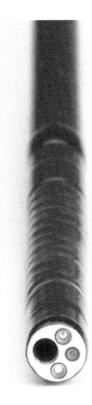

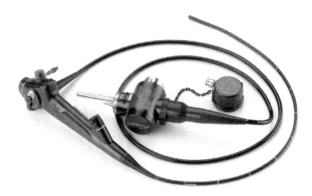

Fig. 1.3 *Distal tip of a video bronchoscope showing the instrument channel, fibreoptics and charge-coupled device video chip.*

Fig. 1.4 *Video bronchoscope with connections to image processor and light source.*

other purposes, i.e. larger instrument channels, dual channels or simply to facilitate the manufacture of slimmer bronchoscopes.

The distal end of the bronchoscope can be rotated through 160° by a lever at the end of the scope. This, in combination with manual rotation of the scope, allows it to be manipulated during examination of the airways. The new range of scopes being developed also have a rotating function with the ability to lock the degree of rotation in a specific position. This development increases the range of movement of the bronchoscope and facilitates access to some of the areas in the lung.

A wide range variety of bronchoscopes are available with different external diameters ranging from 2.2 to 6.3 mm (Fig. 1.5). The instrument channels and the quality of the video chip and images also vary accordingly (Fig. 1.6). A standard bronchoscope should be able to undertake the majority of tasks (good CCD, instrument channel of at least 2.2 mm and external diameter of about 4.6 mm). Slimmer bronchoscopes can allow for smaller airways to be inspected and sampled. An ultra-fine bronchoscope can examine much smaller airways but can also facilitate other procedures such as insertion of stents etc. under direct vision. A larger bronchoscope with a large instrument channel would be more appropriate for interventional procedures where a large channel for suction and introduction of instruments is required. Bronchoscopes with a built-in linear array ultrasound probe are also available which allow sampling of lymph nodes and lung masses adjacent to the central airways (Fig. 1.7).

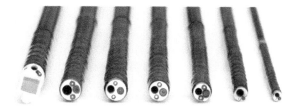

Fig. 1.5 *Distal portion of a number of bronchoscopes showing the variety of instruments available with differing external diameters and functional characteristics.*

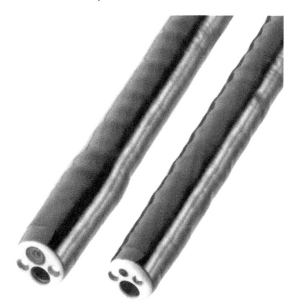

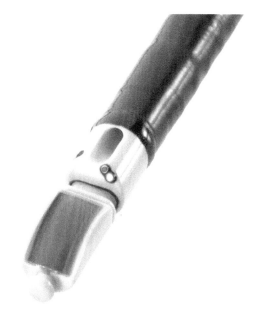

Fig. 1.6 *Two bronchoscopes with different sizes of the charge-coupled device video chip, and instrument channel.*

Fig. 1.7 *Distal tip of the linear array ultrasound bronchoscope.*

Disinfection

Manual cleaning of the bronchoscope is an essential step, as any biological debris left behind would not be adequately sterilized by any disinfectant liquid. The suction parts and instrument channels are susceptible areas where debris may not be completely removed and can then become colonized by bacteria. Manual cleaning with a brush is the most important first step and this is usually followed by automatic disinfection. Instruments are placed in specialized washers and cleaned with disinfection solution such as 0.2 per cent para-acetic acid. The method of disinfecting instruments by hand and placing them in a disinfection solution such as 2 per cent alkaline glutaraldehyde is being phased out due to the risks to staff from occupational exposure to the fumes from the cleaning liquids. Most modern systems can clean several scopes in one cycle and a wash cycle usually lasts 40 minutes.

Cross-infection has been observed with organisms such as environmental *Mycobacterium* and *Pseudomonas* species. Hence processes should be in place to ensure that records of disinfection before use in a patient and the serial numbers of bronchoscopes used in individual patients are maintained. This is essential for tracing patients in the event of suspected cross-infection. Again, in the majority of cases, inadequate manual cleaning of the bronchoscopes, particularly of the suction ports has been a key factor.

Biopsy forceps and needles are more invasive and hence need to be sterilized rather than simply disinfected. The potential risk of infection with viruses and prions has driven the development of single-use disposable instruments. Hence, in most bronchoscopy units, the biopsy forceps, transbronchial aspiration needles and so on are now disposable single-use instruments. Bronchoscopes that can be sterilized rather than disinfected are also in development, which would further reduce the risk from prions, but these would require most bronchoscopy units to significantly increase the number of instruments they have in order to manage a bronchoscopy list. Single-use bronchoscopes are also in development which employ LED light sources and small distal chips within a simple plastic tubing. However, thus far they have limited functionality.

Indications

The main indications for flexible bronchoscopy are listed in Box 1.1. Suspected lung cancer is the major indication for bronchoscopy followed by the assessment of pulmonary infiltrates for microbiological sampling. Traditionally bronchoscopy was conducted for diagnostic purposes but the role of therapeutic bronchoscopy is increasing with the development of new endoscopic treatments for respiratory diseases.

BOX 1.1 Indications for bronchoscopy

- Investigations of symptoms
  - haemoptysis
  - persistent cough
  - recurrent infection

- Suspected neoplasia
  - unexplained paralysis of vocal cords
  - stridor
  - localized monophonic wheeze
  - segmental or lobar collapse
  - assessment of nodules or masses identified on radiology
  - unexplained paralysis of hemi-diaphragm or raised right hemi-diaphragm
  - suspicious sputum cytology
  - unexplained pleural effusions
  - mediastinal tissue diagnosis and staging
  - assess suitability for surgery
  - staging of lung cancer

- Infection
  - assessment of pulmonary infiltrates
  - identification of organisms
  - evaluate airways if recurrent or persistent infection
  - clinical or radiological features of environmental mycobacterial infection

- Diffuse lung disease
  - differential cell counts and cytology
  - transbronchial lung biopsy

- Therapeutic
  - clearance of airway secretions
  - recurrent mucous plugging causing lobar collapse and atelectasis in patients on mechanical ventilators
  - foreign body removal
  - palliation of neoplasm
  - endobronchial ablation of tumour (cryotherapy, electrocautery, laser)
  - insertion of airway stents
  - insertion of brachytherapy catheters
  - insertion of fiducial markers for the gamma/cyberknife
  - bronchoscopic lung volume reduction
  - bronchial thermoplasty for asthma
  - treatment of bronchopleural fistula

Contraindications

Failure of the patient or their representative (in special circumstances) to provide consent is a contraindication, and written consent is required before the procedure. The main contraindications for bronchoscopy are hypoxia that cannot be adequately corrected by oxygen supplementation and a bleeding diathesis. However, even in these circumstances, firm cut-offs are not given as the risk–benefit should be evaluated on an individual-patient basis. Full resuscitation equipment should be available in the bronchoscopy suite and the staff should have the appropriate level of skill and experience to deal with any potential complications. These include respiratory failure, cardiac arrhythmias, haemorrhage and intercostal drain insertion.

Patient preparation

All patients need to provide informed consent prior to the procedure. They should be provided with written information in advance of the procedure and the key aspects, such as risks of the procedure and alternative approaches, should be discussed before final consent. The procedure is usually performed on an outpatient basis with conscious sedation. Patients should be advised not to eat for at least 6 hours before the procedure but they may be allowed to drink water for up to 2 hours before the procedure. Box 1.2 provides a simple checklist for patient preparation prior to the procedure.

BOX 1.2 Preparation for bronchoscopy

- Patient information – verbal and written
- Full blood count and clotting prior to transbronchial lung biopsy and interventional procedures such as tumour ablation
- Informed consent
- Spirometry if oxygen saturations < 95 per cent
- Arterial blood gases if oxygen saturations < 92 per cent
- Baseline electrocardiogram (ECG) if there is a history of cardiac disease
- If patients are to have any sedation, ensure that someone is going to accompany them home after the procedure
- Remind patients that if they are sedated they will be unable to drive or operate machinery for at least 24 hours
- Intravenous access
- Consider bronchodilators if there is evidence of bronchospasm
- Consider prophylactic antibiotics if at very high risk of endocarditis: asplenia, heart valve prosthesis or previous history of endocarditis

---

Computed tomography (CT) scan should be performed prior to bronchoscopy and there is good evidence that reviewing CT scans of the thorax before flexible bronchoscopy significantly improves the yield from the procedure. It allows the bronchoscopist to select more accurately the segment of the lung that should be sampled and hence improve the diagnostic accuracy of the investigation. The CT scan may also demonstrate the presence of mediastinal lymph nodes and hence allow additional procedures such as transbronchial fine-needle aspiration to be performed at the same time as the diagnostic bronchoscopy.

Sedation

Bronchoscopy can be easily performed without any sedation providing the patient is relaxed and fully informed about the procedure and what to expect. Short-acting sedatives that are commonly used include a short-acting intravenous (IV) benzodiazepine, such as IV midazolam, or an opiate such as fentanyl or alfentanil. Midazolam has the advantage of amnesic properties whereas fentanyl or alfentanil have good antitussive properties. In some institutions, low-dose propofol infusion is used to induce and maintain sedation.

Patients who have been given sedation should be advised not to drive or handle any machinery for at least 24 hours after the procedure. Patients who are given sedatives need to be collected and accompanied home after the procedure.

Room ergonomics and approach to the procedure

The procedure can be performed with the patient sitting upright in a semi-recumbent position being approached from the front (Fig. 1.8). This has the advantage of allowing it to be carried out in sicker patients who desaturate upon lying flat. For this setup the bronchoscope image obtained is such that the posterior aspect is visible at the top, the anterior aspect is below, the right is on the left part of the image and the left is on the right part of the image (Fig. 1.9).

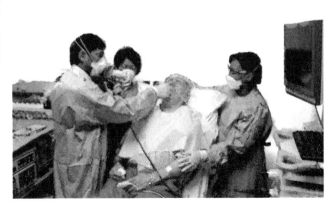

Fig. 1.8 *Room setup with the semi-recumbent patient being approached from the front.*

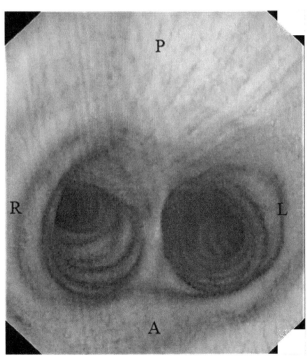

Fig. 1.9 *Bronchoscopic image obtained with the semi-recumbent patient approached from the front.*

The posterior approach with the patient lying flat is also widely used (Fig. 1.10). This approach is also required in a number of procedures such as endobronchial ultrasound and also the superdimension procedure. With this approach the image obtained is such that the anterior aspect is at the top, the posterior aspect is the inferior aspect of the image and the left side of the patient is the left sided image and the right side of the patient is the right side of the image (Fig. 1.11).

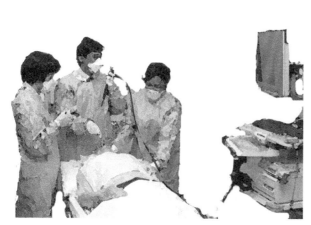

Fig. 1.10 *Room setup with patient being approached from the back in a supine position.*

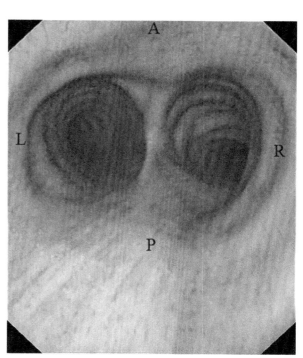

Fig. 1.11 *Bronchoscopic image obtained with the supine patient approached from the back.*

The different approaches have their own merits and limitations and we would advocate that the bronchoscopist becomes familiar with both approaches and hence becomes flexible and adaptive to the circumstances. In order to simplify the anatomy for beginners, this is discussed separately in the following chapters, depending on the approach. Chapter 3 demonstrates the anatomy according to the anterior approach and Chapter 4 the anatomy according to the posterior approach.

Basic techniques and sampling

● *Bronchial washings*

Bronchial washings allow targeted sampling of proximal or segmental airways. The bronchoscope is held proximal, but close, to the site of abnormality. About 10–20 mL aliquots of saline are instilled and aspirated back. The sensitivity of bronchial washings is very variable (average 50 per cent; range 21–76 per cent).

● *Bronchial biopsies*

A variety of biopsy forceps, from cupped to serrated, are available for obtaining tissue samples. The forceps are inserted through the instrument channel of the bronchoscope. The forceps are just opened, apposed to the area of abnormality and then closed in order to obtain biopsies under direct vision (Fig. 1.12). Several biopsies should be obtained to ensure that adequate tissue has been obtained for diagnosis. Crush artefact is the main limiting factor that affects the interpretation of the tissue obtained. A higher yield is obtained from endobronchial biopsies, with an overall sensitivity of 74 (range 48–97) per cent. However, where an exophytic tumour is visible, the diagnostic yield should be at least 90 per cent. The technique is generally very safe and the main complication is that of bleeding, particularly when vascular lesions are sampled. The bleeding is rarely significant and can usually be controlled with conservative measures.

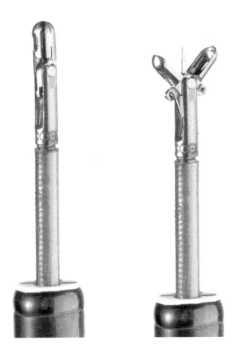

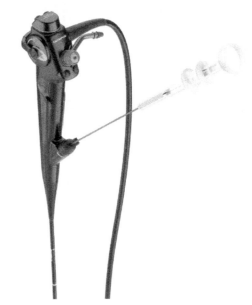

Fig. 1.12a *Distal view of the biopsy forceps in an open and closed position.*

Fig. 1.12b *Proximal view of the biopsy forceps showing the handle that is used to open and shut them.*

● Bronchial brushings

Bronchial brushings can be obtained by using the cytology brush to scrape some cells from the surface of any abnormal areas. The brush consists of fine bristles similar to a bottle brush with a protective plastic sheath. The instrument is passed through the instrument channel of the bronchoscope towards the abnormal area. The brush portion is then protruded out of the plastic sheath and brushed against the abnormal mucosa. The brush is then withdrawn back into the plastic sheath (Fig. 1.13). The cells are then either smeared on to a slide or rinsed into saline according to local preferences. In some centres, the brushings are rinsed into cytolyte solution for processing. The yield from bronchial brushings is 59 (range 23–93) per cent; the main complication is minor bleeding but there is a risk of a pneumothorax where a brush is advanced blindly beyond a subsegmental bronchus.

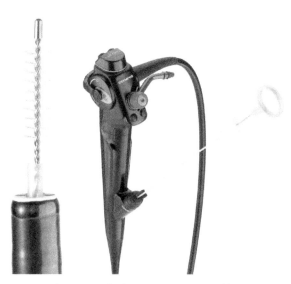

Fig. 1.13a *Close-up of a bronchial brush (left) and handle (right): when the brush is protruding out of the sheath.*

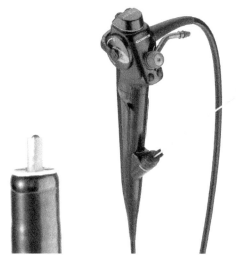

Fig. 1.13b *Close-up of a bronchial brush (left) and handle (right): when the brush is retracted.*

● Bronchoalveolar lavage

Bronchoalveolar lavage enables sampling of the distal airways and alveolar spaces. It is particularly useful in the assessment of:

- diffuse interstitial lung disease
- parenchymal infiltrates
- pulmonary infiltrates in immunocompromised patients
- assessment of occupational dust exposure.

The procedure is performed by wedging the bronchoscope in the desired subsegment. In diffuse lung disease, the right middle lobe is the segment of choice as it drains well and hence provides the best yield. Otherwise the optimal segment is selected on the basis of radiological findings. Once the bronchoscope is wedged into the subsegment, 50–60 mL aliquots of normal saline are instilled and aspirated back either by gentle hand suction or with low-pressure suction into a collecting bottle. The total fluid instilled ranges from 100 to 250 mL depending on the exact indication and local circumstances. The key aspect of the technique is to maintain the position of the bronchoscope in the bronchial segment and also to maintain low suction pressure. Displacement of the bronchoscope and higher suction pressure causing airway collapse are the main factors that lead to lower yields from bronchoalveolar lavage. Patients with obstructive airways disease and emphysema also tend to have low yields. The main adverse events in bronchoalveolar lavage are usually cough, dyspnoea, wheezing and transient fevers. A significant proportion of the patients who are sampled are hypoxic due to underlying disease, and instillation of significant volumes of saline can precipitate hypoxia and in some patients with pulmonary oedema.

The sampling provides information on the cellular composition of the pulmonary infiltrates, types of infective organisms, and presence of particulate and acellular material in the alveolar spaces. Identification of specific bacteria, fungi and acid-fast bacilli may be diagnostic. Malignant cells can be identified in the lavage in patients with bronchioloalveolar cell carcinoma, lymphangitis carcinomatosis or diffuse metastatic disease. Milky proteinaceous lavage which is laden with amorphous periodic acid-Schiff (PAS)-positive staining to the debris is almost pathognomonic of pulmonary alveolar-proteinosis.

Transbronchial lung biopsy

Transbronchial lung biopsy is utilized in the assessment of diffuse lung disease and in patients where there is a localized parenchymal shadow (at least involving a pulmonary segment). The yield is greater in bronchocentric conditions such as sarcoidosis. It also has a useful role in the diagnosis of diffuse lung diseases, such as lymphangitis carcinomatosis, disseminated malignancy, interstitial pneumonitis and extrinsic allergic alveolitis.

The biopsy forceps are inserted through the instrument channel of the bronchoscope into the desired segment. Ideally the bronchoscope should also be wedged into this area, so that if there is any bleeding it can be contained within a small area of the lung. The forceps should be advanced until there is resistance during inspiration. The forceps are then withdrawn 1–2 cm and opened. The patient is then asked to breathe out whilst the forceps are advanced during expiration. When resistance is felt, the forceps are closed and gently tugged. This is usually repeated until four biopsies are obtained for pathological analysis.

The two main adverse events from transbronchial lung biopsy are haemorrhage and pneumothorax. The risk of a pneumothorax is between 5 and 10 per cent, but a clinically significant pneumothorax requiring intervention occurs in about 1 per cent of cases. The degree of bleeding is very variable but blood loss of more than 250 mL is infrequent. Any significant bleeding is managed with suctioning of any blood, combined with instillation of ice-cold saline and diluted adrenaline (1:100000). As described earlier, wedging of the bronchoscope in the segment where the biopsy is obtained also contains the bleeding. For additional information regarding management, please see the section on airway haemorrhage (Chapter 12).

Bronchopulmonary segments

The lungs are made up of the right and left lung, three lobes in the right lung, two lobes in the left lung, 10 segments in the right lung and nine segments in the left lung. The trachea divides into two main bronchi, which in turn divide into the lobar bronchi and then the segmental bronchi. The segmental bronchi continue to divide into smaller airways. The patency of these airways is maintained by the sections of cartilage within the airway. The cartilaginous component of the airway decreases with more progressive divisions of airways and the airways also become progressively narrow.

Chapter 2

Nomenclature

The bronchopulmonary segments are numbered according to the relative position of the origin of segmental bronchi. The bronchial segment that originates at the highest position is labelled 1 (apical segment of the upper lobe); the next bronchial segment that originates is labelled 2, and so on. The bronchial segments are named using Arabic numerals and pulmonary segments with Roman numerals (Figs 2.1a and 2.2a). The bronchial subsegments are subsequently labelled as a, b, c in sequence. In the left lung the labelling is in a clockwise direction, whereas in the right lung the subsegments are labelled in an anticlockwise direction (Figs 2.1b,c and 2.2b,c).

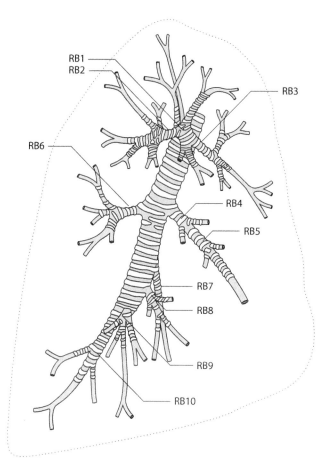

Fig. 2.1a *Right bronchopulmonary tree with numbering of segments.*

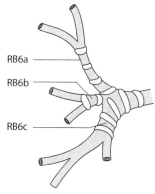

Fig. 2.1b *Example of labelling of subsegments in the right bronchopulmonary tree: segments of the apical segment of the right lower lobe, labelled a, b and c in an anticlockwise direction.*

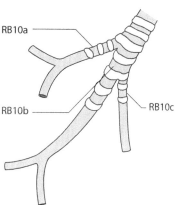

Fig. 2.1c *Example of labelling of subsegments in the right bronchopulmonary tree: segments of the posterior segment of the right lower lobe, labelled a, b and c in an anticlockwise direction.*

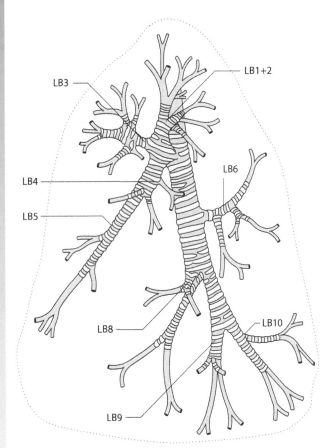

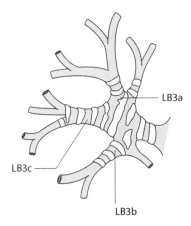

Fig. 2.2a *Left bronchopulmonary tree with numbering of segments.*

Fig. 2.2b *Example of labelling of subsegments in the left bronchopulmonary tree: segments of the anterior segment of the left upper lobe, denoted a, b and c in a clockwise direction.*

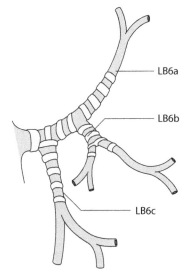

Fig. 2.2c *Example of labelling of subsegments in the left bronchopulmonary tree: segments of the apical segment of the left lower lobe, denoted a, b and c in a clockwise direction.*

The carina are also denoted in a systematic manner. The main carina is labelled as MC. On the right side, the first carina is at the junction of the right upper lobe and the bronchus intermedius (labelled as RC1). The next carina is at the junction of the right middle and the right lower lobe and is labelled as RC2. In the left lung, the main secondary carina is the division between the left upper lobe and the left lower lobe and is termed LC2. The carina between the left upper lobe and the lingula is in a more superior position and is denoted by LC1. Other carina can be denoted according to the segments that form the carina, e.g. the carina between the posterior and anterior segments of the right upper lobe may be described as RC RB2–RB3 (Figs 2.2d–2.2j).

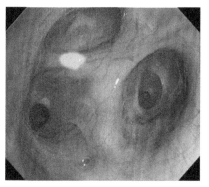

Fig. 2.2d *Highlighted area would be denoted as follows: RC RB1–RB3.*

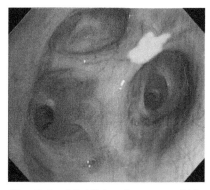

Fig. 2.2e *Highlighted area would be denoted as follows: RC RB1–RB2.*

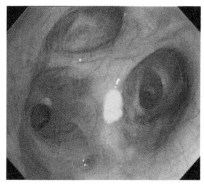

Fig. 2.2f *Highlighted area would be denoted as follows: RC RB2–RB3.*

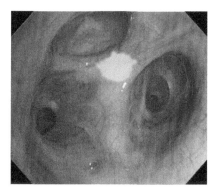

Fig. 2.2g *Highlighted area would be denoted as follows: RC RB1–RB2–RB3.*

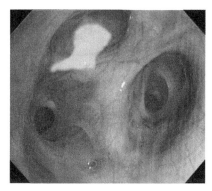

Fig. 2.2h *Highlighted area would be denoted as follows: RB1 to RC RB1–RB3.*

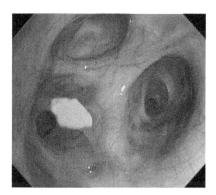

Fig. 2.2i *Highlighted area would be denoted as follows: RB3.*

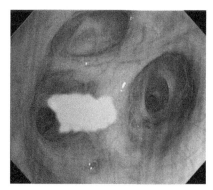

Fig. 2.2j *Highlighted area would be denoted as follows: RB3 to RC RB2–RB3.*

Right lung

The right lung consists of three lobes separated by the oblique and horizontal fissures. The oblique fissure separates the upper and middle lobes from the lower lobes. The horizontal fissure separates the upper and the middle lobes (Fig. 2.3).

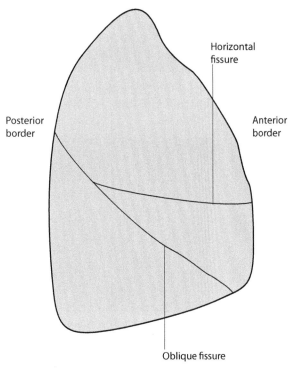

Fig. 2.3a *Oblique and horizontal fissures in the right lung: lateral or costal view.*

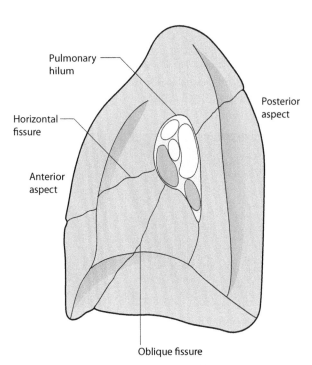

Fig. 2.3b *Oblique and horizontal fissures in the right lung: medial or hilar view.*

● Right upper lobe

The apical segment (RB1) of the right upper lobe is the most superior bronchus from the upper lobe branches. Its branches supply the apical portion of the lung (I). The posterior segment of the right upper lobe is lower (RB2) and branches to form the posteroinferior part of the upper lobe (II). The anterior segment of the right upper lobe is slightly lower (RB3) and branches to form the anterior inferior portion of the upper lobe (III).

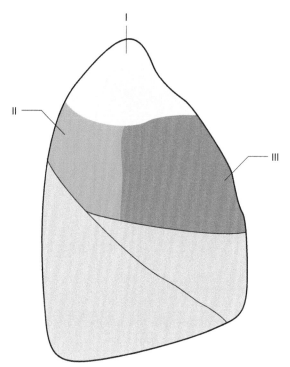

Fig. 2.4a *Apical segments of the lung. I, apical; II, posterior; III, anterior pulmonary segments of the right upper lobe: lateral or costal view.*

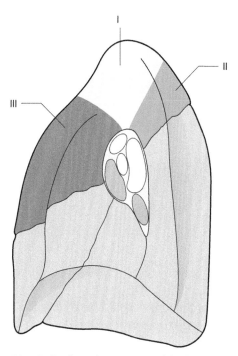

Fig. 2.4b *Apical segments of the lung. I, apical; II, posterior; III, anterior pulmonary segments of the right upper lobe: medial or hilar view.*

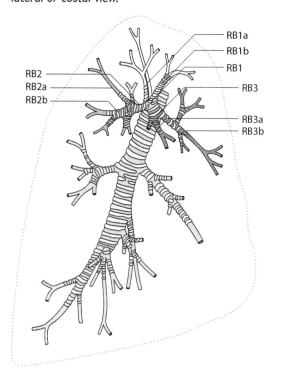

Fig. 2.4c *Right bronchopulmonary tree showing the apical segments of the lung. Right upper lobe: RB1, apical; RB2, posterior; RB3, anterior bronchial segment.*

● *Right middle lobe*

The right middle lobe is a branch from the anterior portion of the right main bronchus. It divides into a lateral segment (RB4) and a medial segment (RB5). These segments form the lateral (IV) and medial portions (V) of the middle lobe.

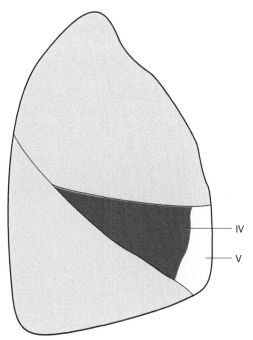

Fig. 2.5a *Segments of the right middle lobe. IV, lateral; V, medial pulmonary segment. Lateral or costal view.*

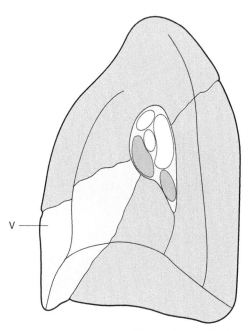

Fig. 2.5b *Segments of the right middle lobe. V, medial pulmonary segment. Medial or hilar view.*

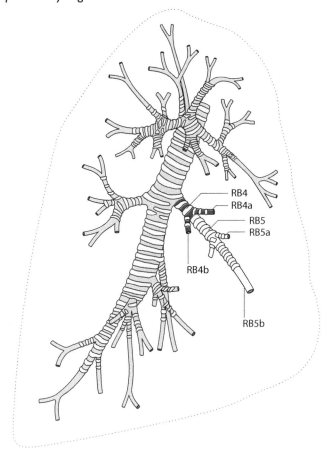

Fig. 2.5c *Right bronchopulmonary tree showing the right middle lobe: RB4, lateral; RB5, medial bronchial segment.*

● Right lower lobe

The right lower lobe bronchus gives off a posterior branch (RB6) a short distance from the right middle lobe origin. This supplies the apical portion to the lower lobe (VI). The main airway continues posterolaterally from its anterior medial aspect to form the origin of the medial segment (RB7), which supplies the inferior medial portion of the lung (VII). It continues to give off the anterior segment (RB8) and supplies the anterior portion of the lower lobe (VIII). The airway continues posterolaterally and also gives off a lateral segment (RB9) and then forms the posterior basal segment (RB10). These form the lateral (IX), and posterior inferior (X) pulmonary segments of the right lung, respectively.

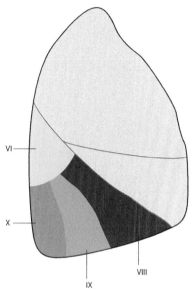

Fig. 2.6a *Basal segments of the right lung. VI, superior; VIII, anterior; IX, lateral; X, posterior pulmonary segments of the right lower lobe. Lateral or costal view.*

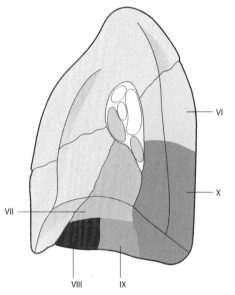

Fig. 2.6b *Basal segments of the right lung. VI, superior; VII, medial; VIII, anterior; IX, lateral; X, posterior pulmonary segments of the right lower lobe. Medial or hilar view.*

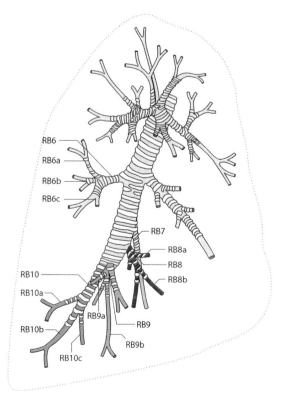

Fig. 2.6c *Right bronchopulmonary tree showing the basal segments. VI, superior; VII, medial; VIII, anterior; IX, lateral; X posterior bronchial segments of the right lower lobe.*

Left lung

The left lung consists of two lobes which are separated by the oblique fissure (Fig. 2.7). The upper lobe comprises five segments and the lower lobe has four segments.

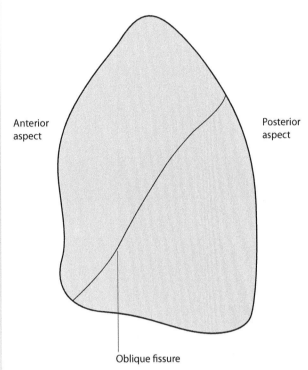

Fig. 2.7a *Oblique fissure of the left lung: lateral or costal view.*

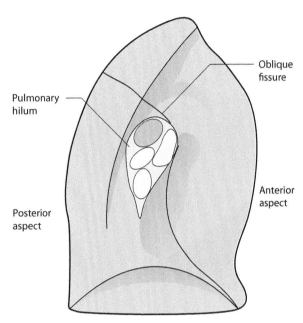

Fig. 2.7b *Oblique fissure of the left lung: medial or hilar view.*

● *Left upper lobe* (Fig. 2.8)

The left upper lobe has a superior and an inferior division. From the superior division, the highest branch is the apicoposterior segment (LB1 + 2), which in turn separates to form the apical segmental bronchus (LB1) and the posterior segmental bronchus (LB2). These form the apical segment (I) and the posterior segment (II) of the upper lobe. Just below the origin of the apicoposterior branch is the anterior branch (LB3) and this forms the anterior segment (III). The inferior division of the left upper lobe forms the lingular segments, the superior branch LB4 forms the superior segment (IV) and the subsequent slightly inferior division (LB5) forms the inferior segment of the lingula (V).

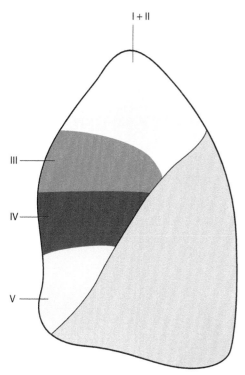

I + II

III

IV

V

Fig. 2.8a *Segments of the upper lobe of the left lung. I + II, apicoposterior; III, anterior ; IV, superior lingular; V, inferior lingular pulmonary segments. Lateral or costal view.*

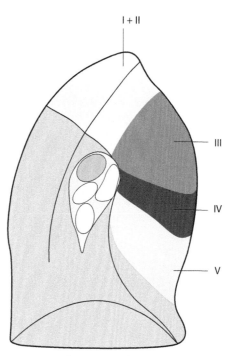

I + II

III

IV

V

Fig. 2.8b *Segments of the upper lobe of the left lung. I + II, apicoposterior; III, anterior ; IV, superior lingular; V, inferior lingular pulmonary segments. Medial or hilar view.*

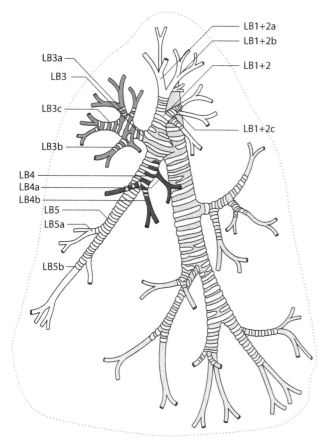

LB1+2a
LB1+2b
LB1+2
LB3a
LB3
LB3c
LB1+2c
LB3b
LB4
LB4a
LB4b
LB5
LB5a
LB5b

Fig. 2.8c *Left bronchopulmonary tree showing the segments of the upper lobe. I + II, apicoposterior; III, anterior; IV, superior lingular; V, inferior lingular bronchial segments.*

● *Left lower lobe* (Fig. 2.9)

The lower lobe bronchus descends in a posterolateral direction. The apical segmental bronchus LB6 arises from the posterior aspect and forms the apical basal lobe (VI). It then gives off an anterior segmental bronchus (LB7 + 8) from its anterior medial aspect to form the anterior basal segment (VIII). The next is the lateral segmental bronchus (LB9) and finally the airway forms the posterior segment of bronchus LB10. The latter two form the lateral aspects of the inferior lobe (IX) and the posteroinferior part of the lower lobe (X).

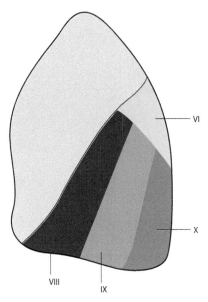

Fig. 2.9a *Basal segments of the lower lobe of the left lung. VI, superior; VIII, anterior; IX, lateral; X, posterior pulmonary segments. Lateral or costal view.*

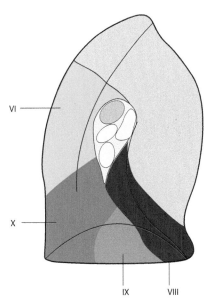

Fig. 2.9b *Basal segments of the lower lobe of the left lung. VI, superior; VIII, anterior; IX, lateral; X, posterior pulmonary segments. Medial or hilar view.*

Fig. 2.9c *Left bronchopulmonary tree showing the basal segments of the left lower lobe. VI, superior; VIII, anterior; IX, lateral; X, posterior bronchial segments.*

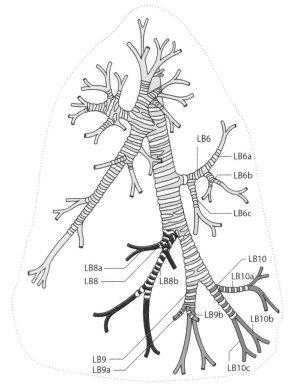

Overall view of segments

The lateral and medial views of the right and left lung, as well as the bronchopulmonary tree, demonstrating all the segments are shown in Figures 2.10 and 2.11.

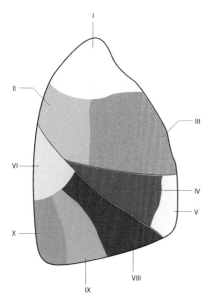

Fig. 2.10a *Segments of the right lung. Right upper lobe: I, apical; II, posterior; III, anterior pulmonary segments. Right middle lobe: IV, lateral; V, medial pulmonary segment. Right lower lobe: VI, superior; VIII, anterior; IX, lateral; X, posterior pulmonary segments. Lateral or costal view.*

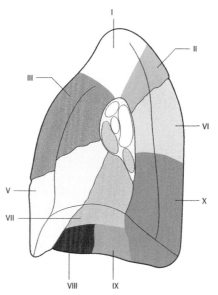

Fig. 2.10b *Segments of the right lung. Right upper lobe: I, apical; II, posterior; III, anterior pulmonary segments. Right middle lobe: IV, lateral; V, medial pulmonary segment. Right lower lobe: VI, superior; VII, medial; VIII, anterior; IX, lateral; X, posterior pulmonary segments. Medial or hilar view.*

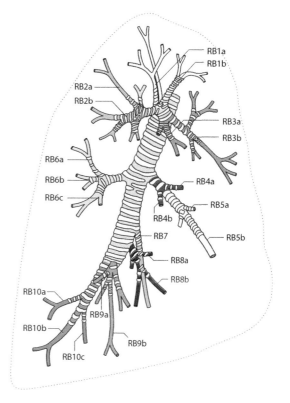

Fig. 2.10c *Right bronchopulmonary tree showing all the segments of the right lung. Right upper lobe: I, apical; II, posterior; III anterior bronchial segments. Right middle lobe: IV, lateral; V, medial bronchial segment. Right lower lobe: VI, superior; VII, medial; VIII, anterior; IX, lateral; X, posterior bronchial segments.*

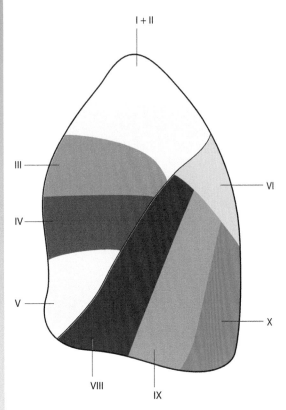

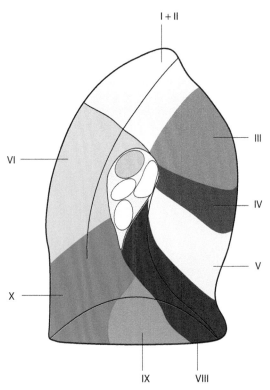

Fig. 2.11a *Segments of the left lung. Left upper lobe: I + II, apicoposterior; III, anterior ; IV, superior lingular; V, inferior lingular pulmonary segments. Left lower lobe: VI, superior; VIII, anterior; IX, lateral; X, posterior pulmonary segments. Lateral or costal view.*

Fig. 2.11b *Segments of the left lung. Left upper lobe: I + II, apicoposterior; III, anterior; IV, superior lingular; V, inferior lingular pulmonary segments. Left lower lobe: VI, superior; VIII, anterior; IX, lateral; X, posterior pulmonary segments. Medial or hilar view.*

Fig. 2.11c *Left bronchopulmonary tree showing all segments of the left lung. Left upper lobe: I + II, apicoposterior; III, anterior ; IV, superior lingular; V, inferior lingular bronchial segments. Left lower lobe: VI, superior; VIII, anterior; IX, lateral; X, posterior bronchial segments.*

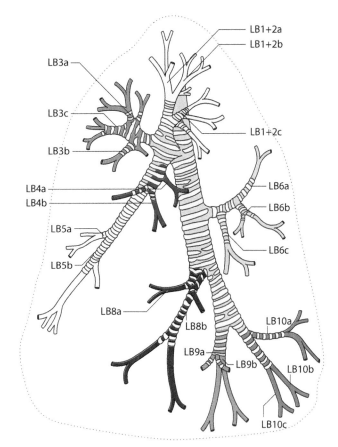

Correlation of CT scans and bronchopulmonary segments

Correlation of the radiographic changes on a computed tomography (CT) scan to a particular bronchopulmonary segment is important and improves the yield from procedures such as bronchial lavage and transbronchial lung biopsy. The images in Figures 2.12–2.17 are to guide the bronchoscopist as to which areas of a CT scan relate to the various bronchopulmonary segments. I also recommend reviewing the whole CT scan carefully and following the airways sequentially to determine the exact segment involved in a particular patient.

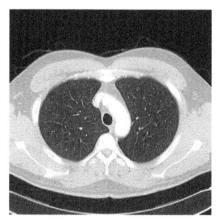

Fig. 2.12a *Cross-sectional CT scans of the thorax at the level of the aortic arch.*

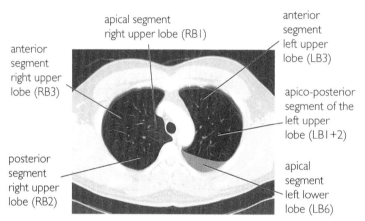

apical segment right upper lobe (RB1)

anterior segment left upper lobe (LB3)

anterior segment right upper lobe (RB3)

apico-posterior segment of the left upper lobe (LB1+2)

posterior segment right upper lobe (RB2)

apical segment left lower lobe (LB6)

Fig. 2.12b *Cross-sectional CT scans of the thorax at the level of the aortic arch; the overlay shows the margins of the pulmonary segments.*

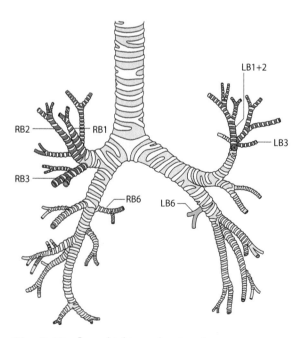

LB1+2

RB2 — RB1

LB3

RB3

RB6   LB6

Fig. 2.12c *Bronchial tree showing the segments correlating with the CT scan.*

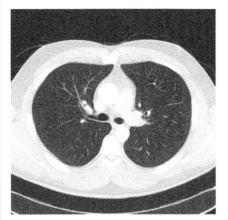

Fig. 2.13a *Cross-sectional CT scans of the thorax at the level of the right upper lobe origin.*

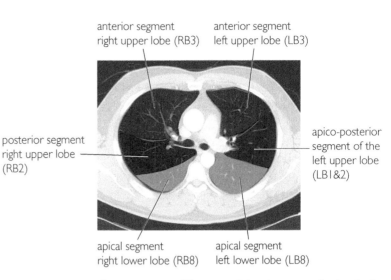

anterior segment right upper lobe (RB3)

anterior segment left upper lobe (LB3)

posterior segment right upper lobe (RB2)

apico-posterior segment of the left upper lobe (LB1&2)

apical segment right lower lobe (RB8)

apical segment left lower lobe (LB8)

Fig. 2.13b *Cross-sectional CT scans of the thorax at the level of the right upper lobe origin; the overlay shows the margins of the pulmonary segments.*

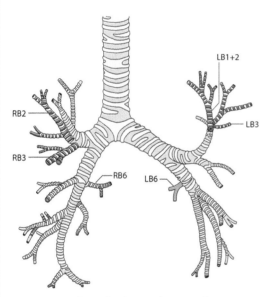

LB1+2

RB2

LB3

RB3

RB6

LB6

Fig. 2.13c *Bronchial tree showing the segments correlating with the CT scan.*

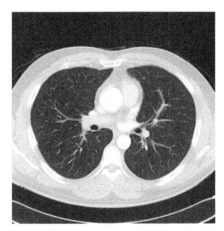

Fig. 2.14a *Cross-sectional CT scans of the thorax at the level of the bronchus intermedius.*

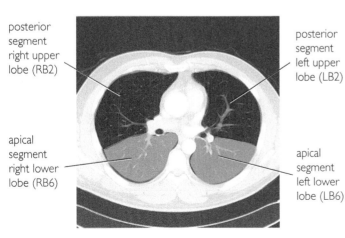

posterior segment right upper lobe (RB2)

posterior segment left upper lobe (LB2)

apical segment right lower lobe (RB6)

apical segment left lower lobe (LB6)

Fig. 2.14b *Cross-sectional CT scans of the thorax at the level of the bronchus intermedius; the overlay shows the margins of the pulmonary segments.*

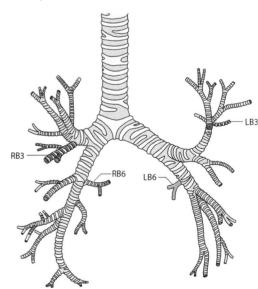

RB3

LB3

RB6

LB6

Fig. 2.14c *Bronchial tree showing the segments correlating with the CT scan.*

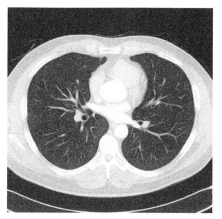

Fig. 2.15a *Cross-sectional CT scans of the thorax at the level of the origin of the right middle lobe.*

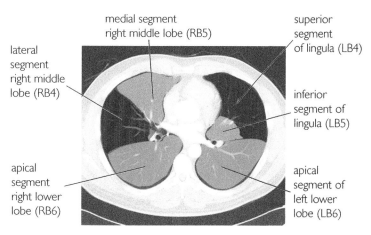

medial segment right middle lobe (RB5)

superior segment of lingula (LB4)

lateral segment right middle lobe (RB4)

inferior segment of lingula (LB5)

apical segment right lower lobe (RB6)

apical segment of left lower lobe (LB6)

Fig. 2.15b *Cross-sectional CT scans of the thorax at the level of the origin of the right middle lobe; the overlay shows the margins of the pulmonary segments.*

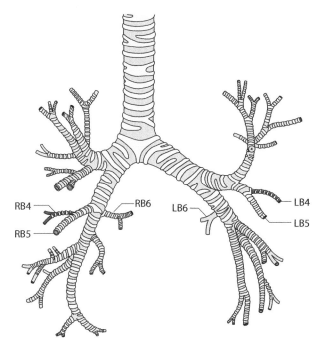

RB4

RB6

LB6

LB4

LB5

RB5

Fig. 2.15c *Bronchial tree showing the segments correlating with the CT scan.*

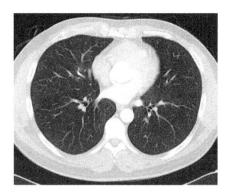

Fig. 2.16a *Cross-sectional CT scans of the thorax at the level of the origin of the lower lobe bronchial segments.*

medial segment of right middle lobe (RB5)

inferior segment of lingula (LB5)

lateral segment of right middle lobe (RB4)

anterior segment of left lower lobe (LB8)

anterior segment of right lower lobe (RB8)

lateral segment of left lower lobe (LB9)

lateral segment of right lower lobe (RB9)

posterior segment of left lower lobe (LB10)

posterior segment of left lower lobe (RB10)

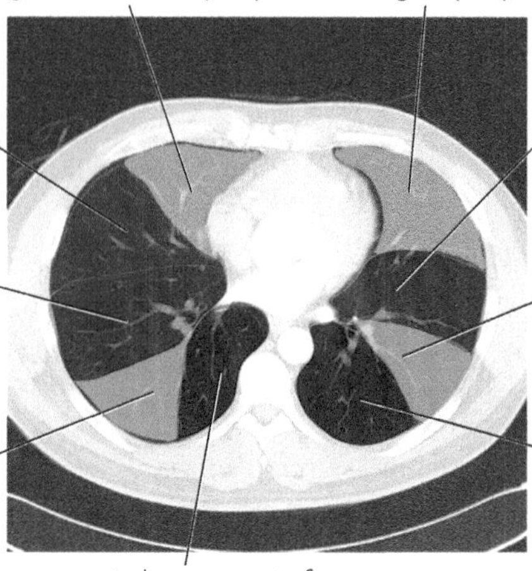

Fig. 2.16b *Cross-sectional CT scans of the thorax at the level of the origin of the lower lobe bronchial segments; the overlay shows the margins of the pulmonary segments.*

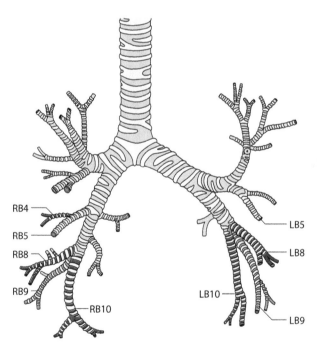

RB4

LB5

RB5

LB8

RB8

RB9

LB10

RB10

LB9

Fig. 2.16c *Bronchial tree showing the segments correlating with the CT scan.*

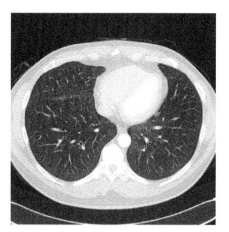

Fig. 2.17a *Cross-sectional CT scans of the thorax at the level of the basal pulmonary segments.*

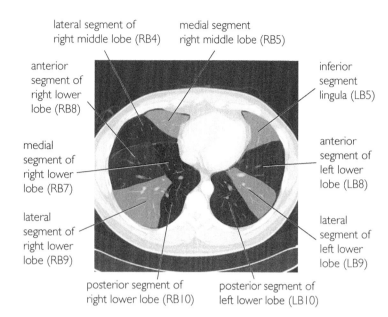

lateral segment of right middle lobe (RB4)

medial segment right middle lobe (RB5)

anterior segment of right lower lobe (RB8)

inferior segment lingula (LB5)

medial segment of right lower lobe (RB7)

anterior segment of left lower lobe (LB8)

lateral segment of right lower lobe (RB9)

lateral segment of left lower lobe (LB9)

posterior segment of right lower lobe (RB10)

posterior segment of left lower lobe (LB10)

Fig. 2.17b *Cross-sectional CT scans of the thorax at the level of the basal pulmonary segments; the overlay shows the margins of the pulmonary segments.*

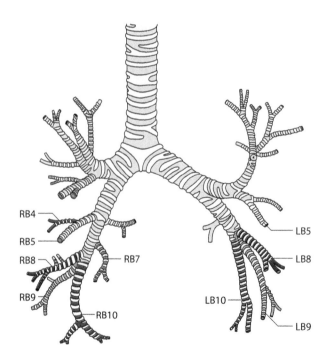

RB4
RB5
RB8 — RB7
RB9
RB10

LB5
LB8
LB10
LB9

Fig. 2.17c *Bronchial tree showing the segments correlating with the CT scan.*

CHAPTER 3

Normal anatomy (anterior approach)

In this chapter the endoscopic images are related to the computed tomography (CT) images. The overall appearance, main characteristics and normal variations are described. The anatomical images in this chapter are presented as they appear when the procedure is performed with the patient in a semi-recumbent position being approached from the front.

In order to minimize confusion, the normal anatomy is described again in the next chapter but the bronchoscopic images are presented as they appear when the patient is bronchoscoped in a supine position and approached from behind.

Vocal cords (Fig. 3.1)

The larynx is composed of a series of cartilages, ligaments and fibrous membranes. At bronchoscopy the epiglottis is the more proximal structure. It is a broad leaf-like structure. The sides are attached by the arytenoid cartilages. The cuneiform and corniculate can be seen at the end of the arytenoid cartilage. The cuneiform cartilage is more anterior and superior to the corniculate cartilage. The vocal folds consist of the false cords or vestibular folds and the true vocal folds. They stretch back from the thyroid angle to the vocal processes of the arytenoids. The vocal folds are involved in the production of sound.

left vocal cord   aryepiglottic fold

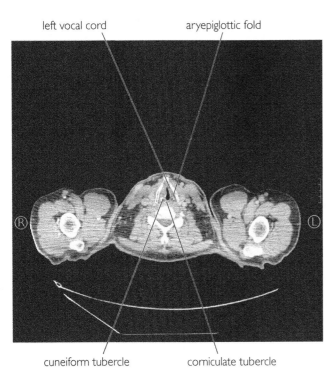

cuneiform tubercle   corniculate tubercle

vocal fold   hyoid bone   cricoid cartilage

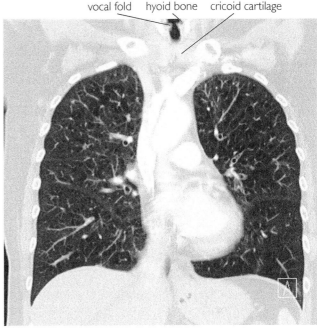

Fig. 3.1a *Cross-sectional CT scan at the superior aspect of the thorax at the level of the vocal cords, which are apposed.*

Fig. 3.1b *Coronal section CT scan of the vocal cords, which are apposed.*

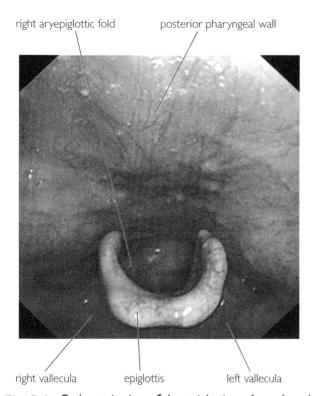

right aryepiglottic fold   posterior pharyngeal wall

right vallecula   epiglottis   left vallecula

Fig. 3.1c *Endoscopic view of the epiglottis and vocal cords.*

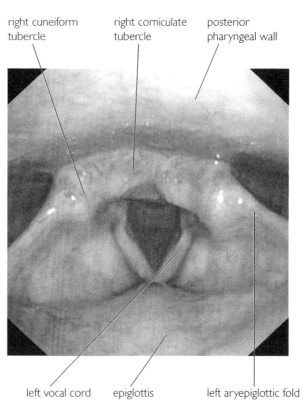

right cuneiform tubercle   right corniculate tubercle   posterior pharyngeal wall

left vocal cord   epiglottis   left aryepiglottic fold

Fig. 3.1d *Endoscopic view of the vocal cords.*

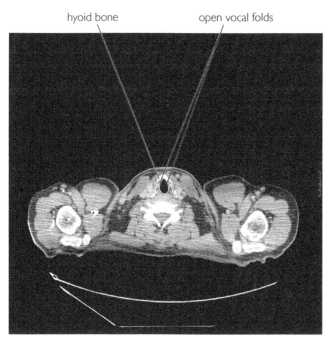

hyoid bone   open vocal folds

Fig. 3.1e *Cross-sectional CT scan at the superior aspect of the thorax at the level of the vocal cords, which are open.*

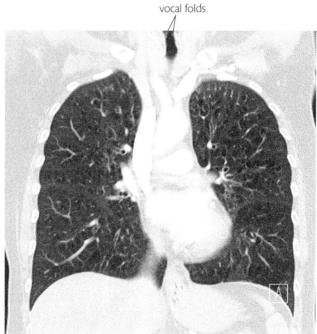

vocal folds

Fig. 3.1f *Coronal section CT scan of the vocal cords, which are open.*

open vocal cords

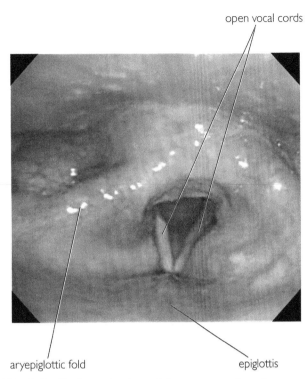

aryepiglottic fold   epiglottis

Fig. 3.1g *Endoscopic view of the open vocal cords.*

corniculate tubercle   apposed vocal cords

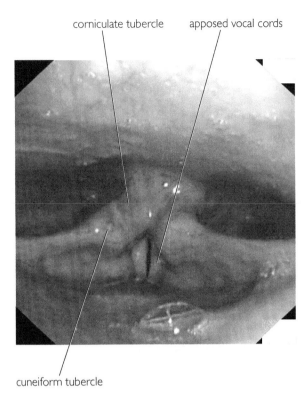

cuneiform tubercle

Fig. 3.1h *Endoscopic view of apposed vocal cords.*

Trachea (Fig. 3.2)

The trachea is a horseshoe- or D-shaped structure which extends from the cricoid cartilage to the carina. The anterior aspect is composed of 16–20 incomplete cartilage rings with a flat fibromuscular posterior component. There is also a longitudinal band of connective tissue which runs down the posterior end of the cartilage. At bronchoscopy the cartilage bands on the anterior surface appear as ridges and the posterior wall appears to bulge into the trachea. The posterior bulge is accentuated in expiration.

The trachea measures approximately 110 mm in length with an external diameter that ranges from 15 mm in women to 20 mm in men. The internal diameter of the trachea is about 12–14 mm.

The trachea divides into the right and left main bronchi at the level of the sternomanubrial junction or the body of the fourth thoracic vertebrae.

A tracheal bronchus is a rare normal variant and originates from the lateral wall of the trachea and into the upper lobe on the right side in about 0.1–2 per cent of individuals and on the left side in 0.3–1 per cent of individuals. The term tracheal bronchus is also used for other anomalous airways arising from the main bronchi and directed to the upper lobes.

superior vena cava   fat   aorta

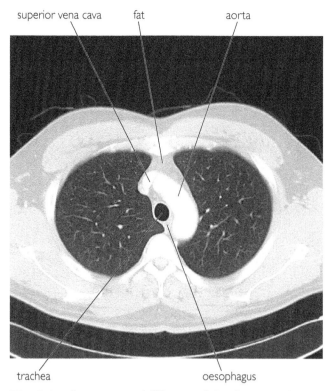

trachea   oesophagus

Fig. 3.2a *Cross-sectional CT scan of the thorax at the mid-tracheal level.*

right pulmonary artery   trachea   aortic arch   left pulmonary artery

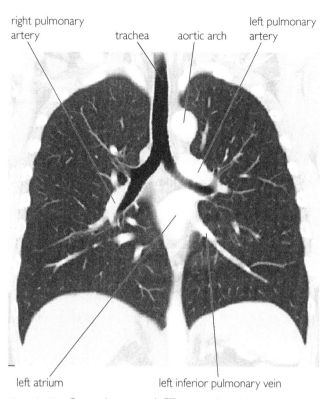

left atrium   left inferior pulmonary vein

Fig. 3.2b *Coronal sectional CT scan of the thorax through the trachea.*

posterior membranous trachea

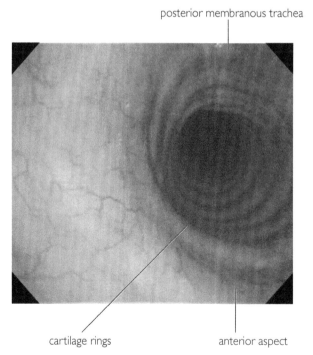

cartilage rings   anterior aspect

Fig. 3.2c *Endoscopic view of the trachea from the level of the subglottis.*

carina   posterior tracheal wall

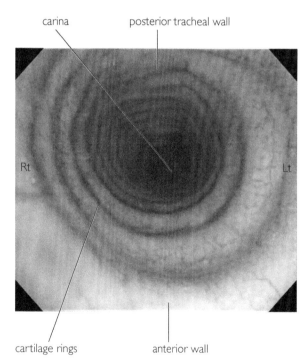

Rt   Lt

cartilage rings   anterior wall

Fig. 3.2d *Endoscopic view of the upper trachea.*

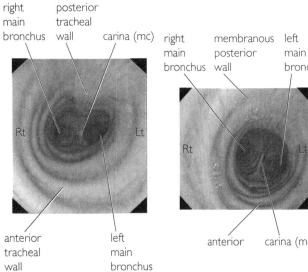

right main bronchus · posterior tracheal wall · carina (mc)

Rt · Lt

anterior tracheal wall · left main bronchus

Fig. 3.2e *Endoscopic view of the trachea from the mid-tracheal level.*

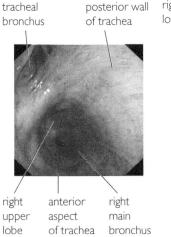

right main bronchus · membranous posterior wall · left main bronchus

Rt · Lt

anterior · carina (mc)

Fig. 3.2f *Endoscopic view of the distal portion of the trachea.*

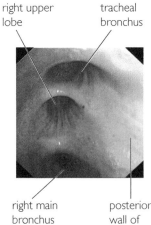

tracheal bronchus · posterior wall of trachea

right upper lobe · anterior aspect of trachea · right main bronchus

Fig. 3.2g *Endoscopic view of a tracheal bronchus as viewed from above with the patient upright and approached from the front. The right upper lobe arises from the right main bronchus.*

right upper lobe · tracheal bronchus

right main bronchus · posterior wall of trachea

Fig. 3.2h *Endoscopic view of a tracheal bronchus as seen at the distal trachea just above the carina. The right upper lobe and bronchus intermedius are visible below.*

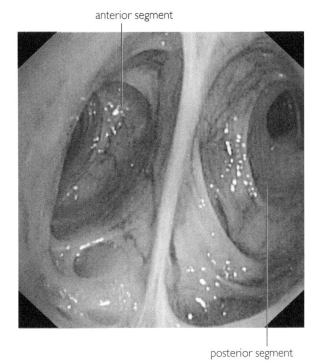

anterior segment

posterior segment

Fig. 3.2i *Bipartite division of the upper lobe in the presence of a tracheal bronchus.*

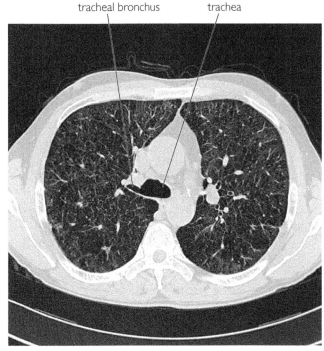

tracheal bronchus · trachea

Fig. 3.2j *Cross-sectional CT scan showing the tracheal bronchus arising at the distal trachea just above the carina.*

Carina (Fig. 3.3)

The carina is a concave spur of cartilage located where the distal trachea divides into the right and left main bronchi. The carina normally appears as a sharp structure and forms the medial borders of the origin of the right and left main bronchi. The sharp angle is maintained as it is primarily composed of cartilage (carinal) and ligaments (interbronchial). Enlargement of the subcarinal structures, such as the subcarinal lymph nodes or the left atrium, may lead to blunting or widening of the carina. It usually measures about 12 mm in diameter and stretches in the midline in the anteroposterior dimension. Very rarely there is an accessory bronchus opening from the lateral walls directed towards the upper lobe.

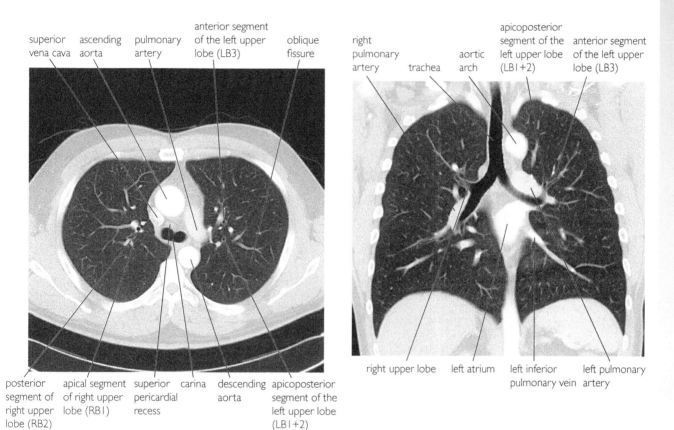

Fig. 3.3a *Cross-sectional CT scan of the thorax at the level of the carina.*

Fig. 3.3b *Coronal sectional CT scan of the thorax through the trachea.*

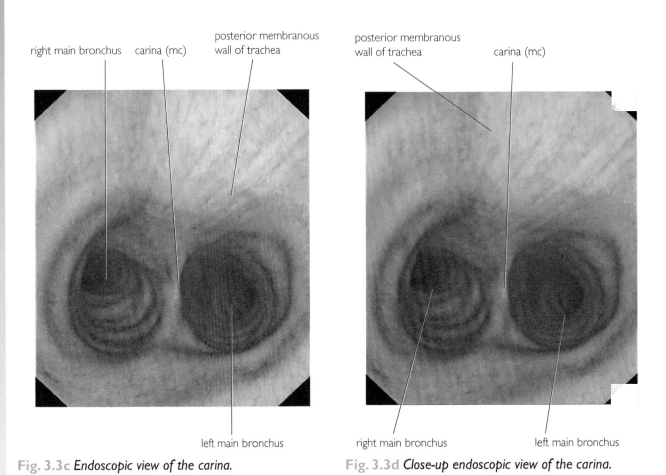

right main bronchus   carina (mc)   posterior membranous wall of trachea

posterior membranous wall of trachea   carina (mc)

left main bronchus

right main bronchus   left main bronchus

Fig. 3.3c *Endoscopic view of the carina.*

Fig. 3.3d *Close-up endoscopic view of the carina.*

Right main bronchus (Fig. 3.4)

The right main bronchus extends from the carina to the origin of the right upper lobe. It then forms the bronchus intermedius. The right main bronchus has a steeper decline from the trachea and hence, in the upright position, foreign bodies tend to fall into the right main bronchus. It is slightly larger in diameter than the left main bronchus, measuring between 10 and 12 mm in external diameter. The inferior lip of the upper lobe bronchus is easily visible at the distal end of the right main bronchus. A rare variation is the origin of an airway leading to the upper lobe. This is classified as a pre-eparterial tracheal bronchus. It may be either a supernumerary or a displaced airway. Where the airway is displaced, there is also a missing upper lobe branch. An accessory cardiac bronchus is a supernumerary bronchus arising from the medial aspect of the right main bronchus and leading towards the pericardium.

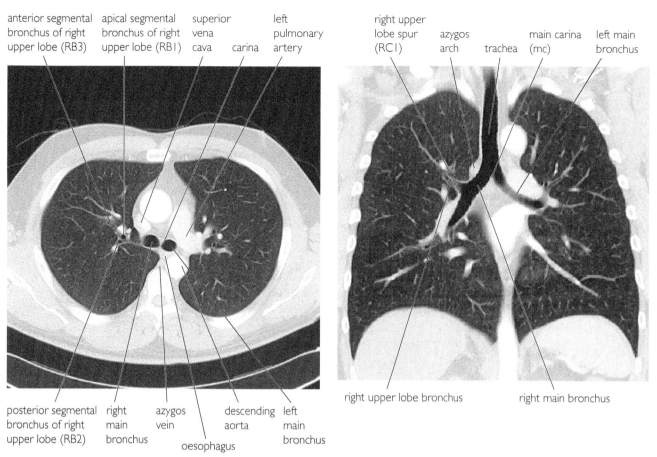

anterior segmental bronchus of right upper lobe (RB3) apical segmental bronchus of right upper lobe (RB1) superior vena cava carina left pulmonary artery

posterior segmental bronchus of right upper lobe (RB2) right main bronchus azygos vein oesophagus descending aorta left main bronchus

Fig. 3.4a *Cross-sectional CT scan of the thorax at the carina, showing the right main bronchus.*

right upper lobe spur (RC1) azygos arch trachea main carina (mc) left main bronchus

right upper lobe bronchus right main bronchus

Fig. 3.4b *Coronal sectional CT scan of the thorax showing the right main bronchus.*

right upper lobe posterior wall of right main bronchus

right upper lobe spur (RC1) bronchus intermedius anterior wall of right main bronchus medial wall of right main bronchus

Fig. 3.4c *Endoscopic view of the right main bronchus visible below the carina.*

right upper lobe origin basal segments posterior wall of right main bronchus

right upper lobe spur (RC1) right middle lobe anterior wall of right main bronchus medial wall of right main bronchus

Fig. 3.4d *Endoscopic view of the right main bronchus with more of the right upper lobe visible.*

Right upper lobe (Fig. 3.5)

The right upper lobe has three main segmental divisions: the apical, anterior and posterior segments. The upper lobe segments divide into segments about 10 mm from the origin. The upper lobe is subject to considerable normal variation:

- In 40 per cent the segmental bronchi arise independently.
- In 24 per cent there is a common apical and anterior trunk and an independent posterior-segmental bronchus. (see Fig. 3.5g)
- In 14 per cent there is a common apical and posterior trunk and an independent anterior segment. (see Fig 3.5h)
- In 10 per cent there is a common anterior and posterior trunk with an independent apical segment.
- In 10 per cent the posterior segmental bronchus is absent.
- In 2 per cent the apical segment is absent.
- In < 1 per cent of patients there is a tracheal bronchus which originates either directly from the trachea or at the level of the carina. In some cases there is an additional branch to the upper lobe, which originates from the right main bronchus.

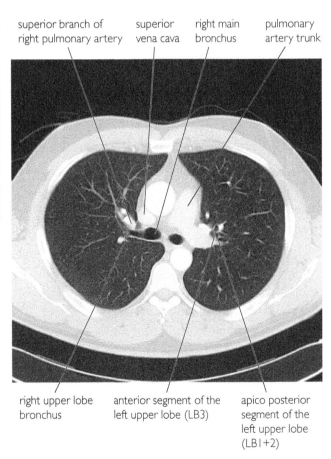

superior branch of right pulmonary artery · superior vena cava · right main bronchus · pulmonary artery trunk

right upper lobe bronchus · anterior segment of the left upper lobe (LB3) · apico posterior segment of the left upper lobe (LB1+2)

Fig. 3.5a *Cross-sectional CT scan of the thorax at the level of the right upper lobe origin.*

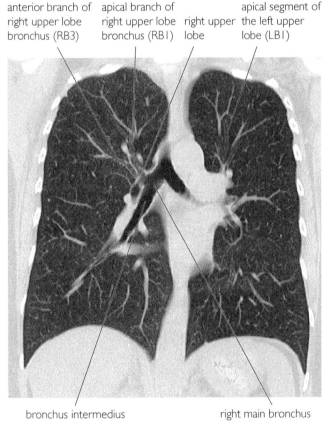

anterior branch of right upper lobe bronchus (RB3) · apical branch of right upper lobe bronchus (RB1) · right upper lobe · apical segment of the left upper lobe (LB1)

bronchus intermedius · right main bronchus

Fig. 3.5b *Coronal sectional CT scan of the thorax showing the right upper lobe.*

apical segment of the
right upper lobe (RB1)   RB2b   RB2a

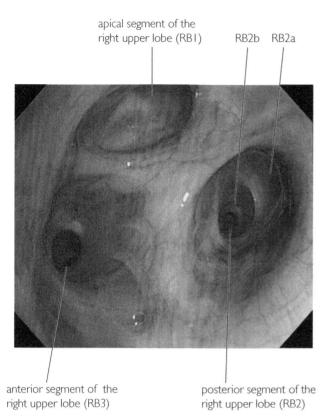

anterior segment of the
right upper lobe (RB3)

posterior segment of the
right upper lobe (RB2)

Fig. 3.5c *Endoscopic view of the right upper lobe from above with the patient upright being approached from the front.*

apical segment of the
right upper lobe (RB1)

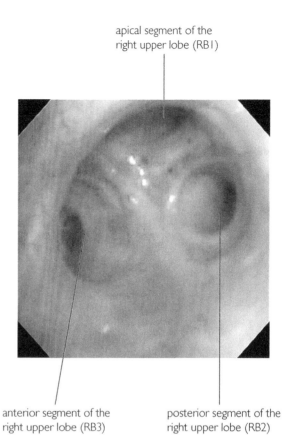

anterior segment of the
right upper lobe (RB3)

posterior segment of the
right upper lobe (RB2)

Fig. 3.5d *Another example of the tripartite right upper lobe arrangement.*

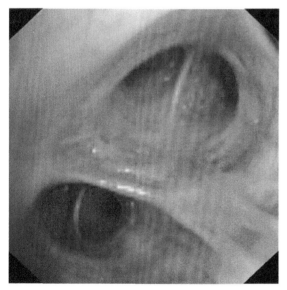

Fig. 3.5e *Bipartite division of the right upper lobe with division at the horizontal axis.*

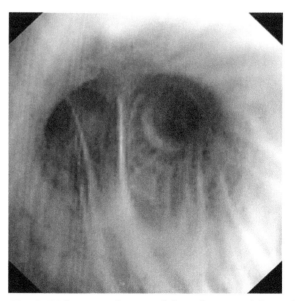

Fig. 3.5f *Bipartite division of the right upper lobe with division in the vertical axis.*

apicoanterior segment of
the right upper lobe (RBI+3)　　　apical segment (RBI)

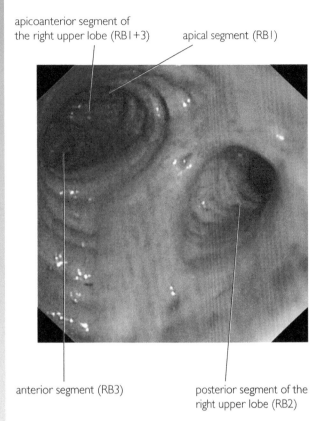

anterior segment (RB3)　　　posterior segment of the
　　　　　　　　　　　　　right upper lobe (RB2)

Fig. 3.5g *Bipartite division of the right upper lobe with apical and anterior segments (RBI + 3 arising together) and a separate posterior segment (RB2).*

apicoposterior segment
anterior segment of the　　of the right upper lobe　　apical segment
right upper lobe (RB3)　　(RBI+2)　　　　　　　　　(RBI)

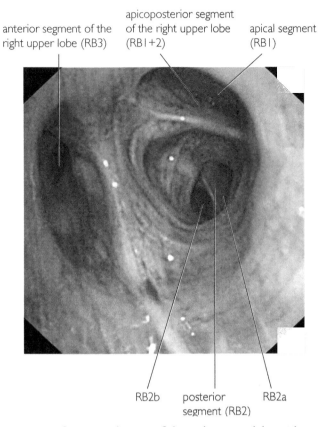

RB2b　　posterior　　RB2a
　　　segment (RB2)

Fig. 3.5h *Bipartite division of the right upper lobe with apical and posterior segments arising together (RBI + 2) and a separate posterior segment (RB3).*

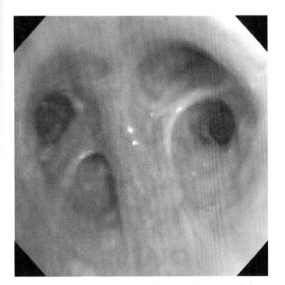

Fig. 3.5i *Four divisions of the right upper lobe.*

Bronchus intermedius (Fig. 3.6)

The bronchus intermedius originates from the right main bronchus and extends from the origin of the right upper lobe to the right middle lobe. It is approximately 20 mm long and has a diameter of about 10 mm. The right middle lobe, the apical segment of the lower lobe and the basal segments are visible at the distal end of bronchus intermedius.

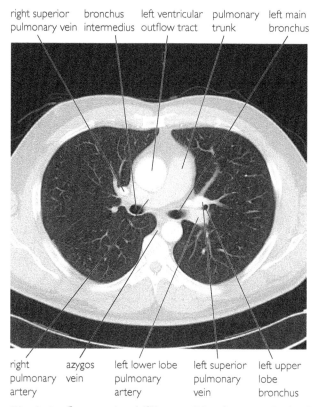

right superior pulmonary vein   bronchus intermedius   left ventricular outflow tract   pulmonary trunk   left main bronchus

right pulmonary artery   azygos vein   left lower lobe pulmonary artery   left superior pulmonary vein   left upper lobe bronchus

Fig. 3.6a *Cross-sectional CT scan of the thorax at the level of the bronchus intermedius (distal to the right upper lobe origin).*

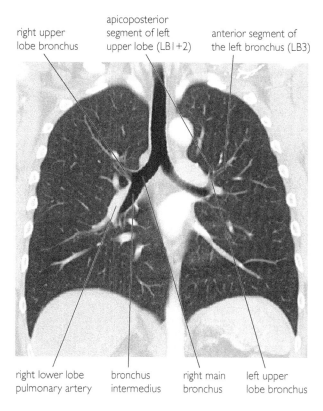

right upper lobe bronchus   apicoposterior segment of left upper lobe (LB1+2)   anterior segment of the left bronchus (LB3)

right lower lobe pulmonary artery   bronchus intermedius   right main bronchus   left upper lobe bronchus

Fig. 3.6b *Coronal sectional CT scan of the thorax through the bronchial tree showing the bronchus intermedius.*

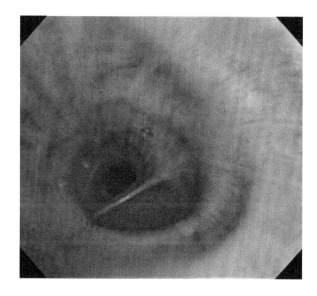

Fig. 3.6c *Endoscopic view of the bronchus intermedius.*

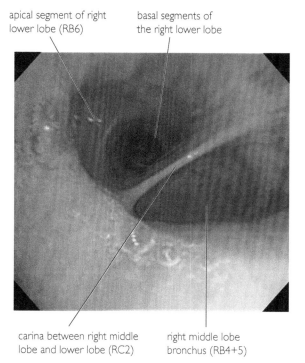

apical segment of right lower lobe (RB6)   basal segments of the right lower lobe

carina between right middle lobe and lower lobe (RC2)   right middle lobe bronchus (RB4+5)

Fig. 3.6d *Endoscopic view of the distal aspect of the bronchus intermedius.*

Right middle lobe (Fig. 3.7)

The right middle lobe is a semi-lunar (D-shaped) bronchus at the anterior end of the bronchus intermedius. In approximately 70 per cent of cases, there are two distinct segments: lateral and medial. In 23 per cent of normal individuals the middle lobe bifurcates in a superior-inferior fashion, similar to that of the lingula. In up to 20 per cent of individuals there is a main lateral bronchus and a smaller medial bronchus which arises from the lateral segment. Occasionally the reverse is seen, with a larger medial segment and a smaller lateral segment arising from it.

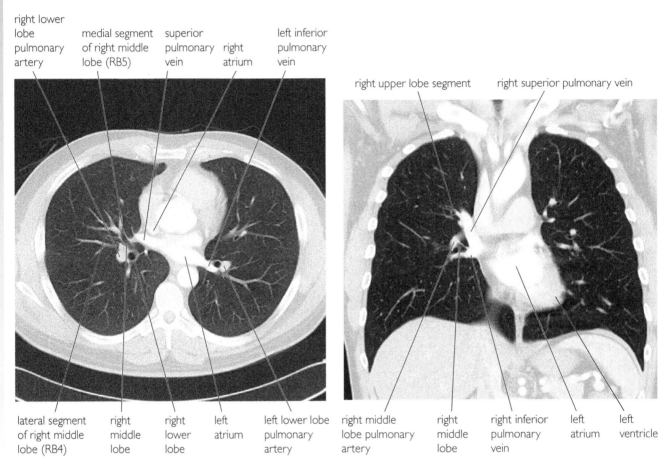

Fig. 3.7a *Cross-sectional CT scan of the thorax at the level of the right middle lobe.*

Fig. 3.7b *Coronal sectional CT scan of the thorax at the level of the right middle lobe.*

basal segments of the
right lower lobe

medial segment of the
right lower lobe (RB7)

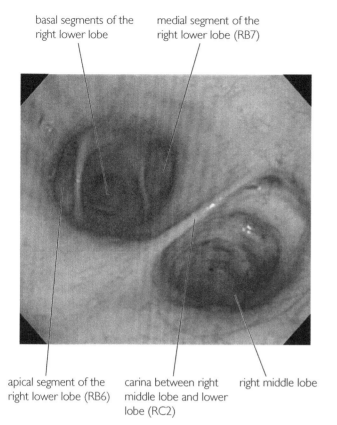

apical segment of the
right lower lobe (RB6)

carina between right
middle lobe and lower
lobe (RC2)

right middle lobe

Fig. 3.7c *Endoscopic view of the right middle and lower lobes.*

right lower lobe segments

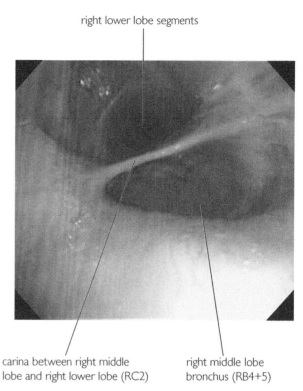

carina between right middle
lobe and right lower lobe (RC2)

right middle lobe
bronchus (RB4+5)

Fig. 3.7d *Endoscopic view of right middle lobe.*

RB4a

lateral segment of the
right lower lobe (RB4)

RB4b

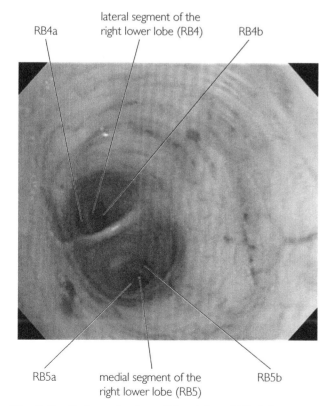

RB5a

medial segment of the
right lower lobe (RB5)

RB5b

Fig. 3.7e *Endoscopic view of the right middle lobe subsegments viewed from the origin of the right middle lobe bronchus.*

RB4a

lateral segment of the
right middle lobe (RB4)

RB4b

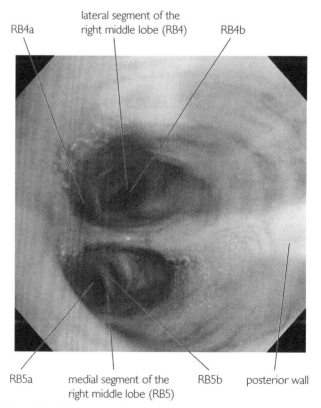

RB5a

medial segment of the
right middle lobe (RB5)

RB5b

posterior wall

Fig. 3.7f *Close-up endoscopic view of the right middle lobe subsegments.*

Right lower lobe (Fig. 3.8)

The right lower lobe comprises five main segments: apical basal, medial basal, anterior basal, lateral basal and posterior basal. In about 40–60 per cent of individuals there is an additional subapical basal segment. The apical basal segment of the right lower lobe is positioned posteriorly at the end of the bronchus intermedius. The apical segment divides immediately into three subsegmental bronchi. The normal pattern observed in the lower lobe bronchial segments are a large medial basal segment (RB7), which is proximal to the other basal segments. The anterior basal segment is in the lateral position, with the lower bronchus dividing further into lateral and posterior segments. This pattern is seen in over 70 per cent of individuals. The other common variation observed is where the anterior basal, lateral basal and posterior basal segments all originate independently at the same level.

A bipartite division is occasionally observed where the anterior and lateral segments arise together proximally to the posterior basal segment from a separate branch. The position and size of the apical basal segment frequently influence the pattern of branching of the basal segments. For example, in some individuals there is a larger apical bronchus and, as a result, the medial through to posterior segment arises in a tripartite from the same level.

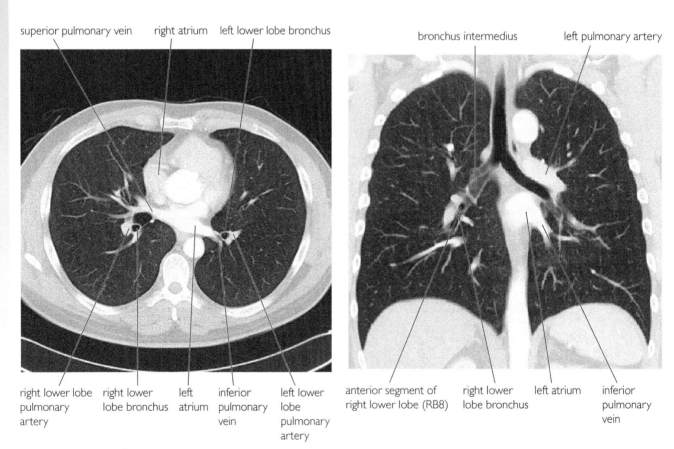

Fig. 3.8a *Cross-sectional CT scan of the thorax at the level of the basal segments of the right lower lobe.*

Fig. 3.8b *Coronal sectional CT scan showing the right lower lobe.*

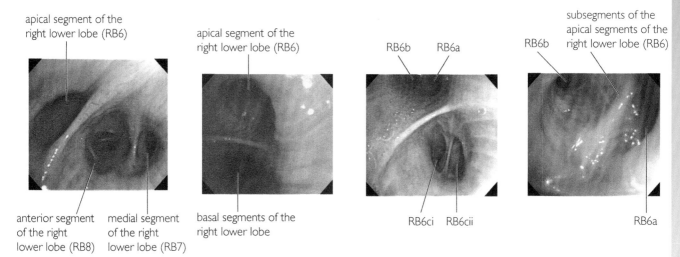

apical segment of the
right lower lobe (RB6)

apical segment of the
right lower lobe (RB6)

RB6b   RB6a

subsegments of the
apical segments of the
RB6b   right lower lobe (RB6)

anterior segment   medial segment
of the right   of the right
lower lobe (RB8)   lower lobe (RB7)

basal segments of the
right lower lobe

RB6ci   RB6cii

RB6a

Fig. 3.8c *Endoscopic view
of the basal segments of the
right lower lobe.*

Fig. 3.8d *Endoscopic view
of the right apicobasal
segment.*

Fig. 3.8e *Endoscopic view
of the apicobasal segments
of the right lower lobe.*

Fig. 3.8f *Close-up
endoscopic view of the right
apicobasal subsegments.*

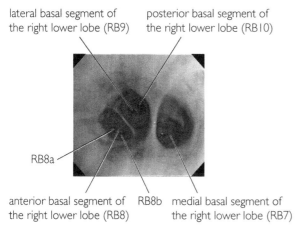

lateral basal segment of
the right lower lobe (RB9)

posterior basal segment of
the right lower lobe (RB10)

RB8a

anterior basal segment of   RB8b   medial basal segment of
the right lower lobe (RB8)   the right lower lobe (RB7)

Fig. 3.8g *Endoscopic view of the basal segments of
the right lower lobe.*

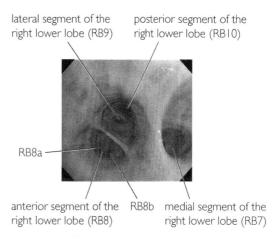

lateral segment of the
right lower lobe (RB9)

posterior segment of the
right lower lobe (RB10)

RB8a

anterior segment of the   RB8b   medial segment of the
right lower lobe (RB8)   right lower lobe (RB7)

Fig. 3.8h *Closer endoscopic view of the basal
segments of the right lower lobe.*

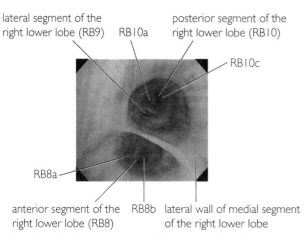

lateral segment of the
right lower lobe (RB9)   RB10a

posterior segment of the
right lower lobe (RB10)

RB10c

RB8a

anterior segment of the   RB8b   lateral wall of medial segment
right lower lobe (RB8)   of the right lower lobe

Fig. 3.8i *Endoscopic view of the anterobasal,
basolateral and posterobasal segments of the right
lower lobe.*

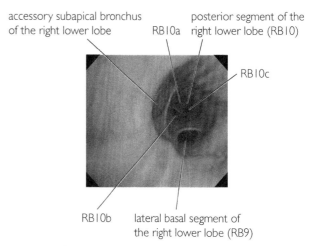

accessory subapical bronchus
of the right lower lobe   RB10a

posterior segment of the
right lower lobe (RB10)

RB10c

RB10b   lateral basal segment of
the right lower lobe (RB9)

Fig. 3.8j *Endoscopic view of the basolateral and
posterobasal segments of the right lower lobe. In this
example a normal variant subapical segment is present.*

anterior segment right
lower lobe (RB8)

inferior pulmonary vein

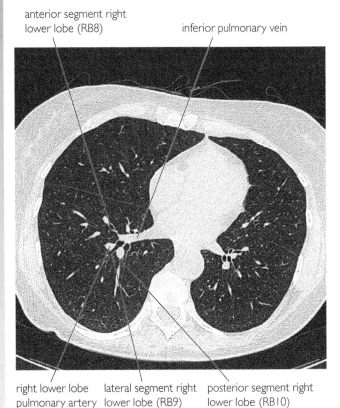

right lower lobe   lateral segment right   posterior segment right
pulmonary artery   lower lobe (RB9)   lower lobe (RB10)

Fig. 3.8k *Cross-sectional CT scan at the level of the basal segments of the right lower lobe.*

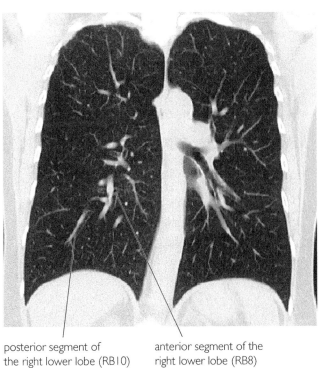

posterior segment of   anterior segment of the
the right lower lobe (RB10)   right lower lobe (RB8)

Fig. 3.8l *Coronal CT scan showing the basal segments of the right lower lobe.*

lateral segment of
the right lower lobe (RB9)

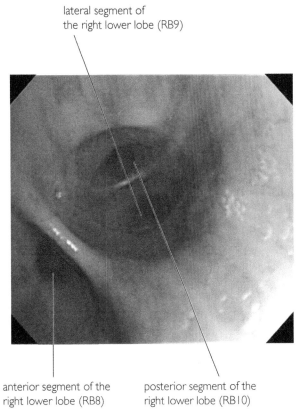

anterior segment of the   posterior segment of the
right lower lobe (RB8)   right lower lobe (RB10)

Fig. 3.8m *Endoscopic view of the anterobasal, basolateral and posterobasal segments of the right lower lobe.*

accessory subapical segment
of the right lower lobe

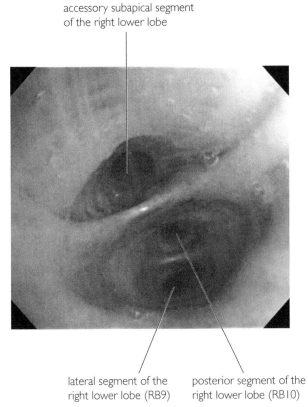

lateral segment of the   posterior segment of the
right lower lobe (RB9)   right lower lobe (RB10)

Fig. 3.8n *Endoscopic view of the basolateral and posterobasal segments of the right lower lobe.*

lateral segment of the right lower lobe (RB9)

accessory subapical segment of the right lower lobe

posterior segment of the right lower lobe (RB10)

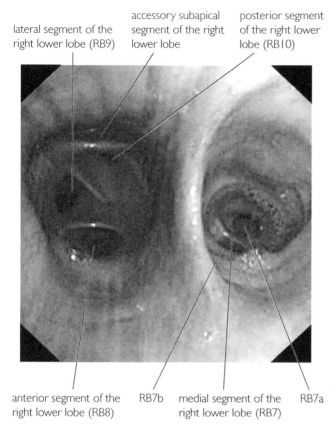

anterior segment of the right lower lobe (RB8)

RB7b

medial segment of the right lower lobe (RB7)

RB7a

Fig. 3.8o *Endoscopic view of the basal segments of the right lower lobe showing a normal variant of a subapical segment.*

lateral segment of the right lower lobe (RB9)

posterior segment of the right lower lobe (RB10)

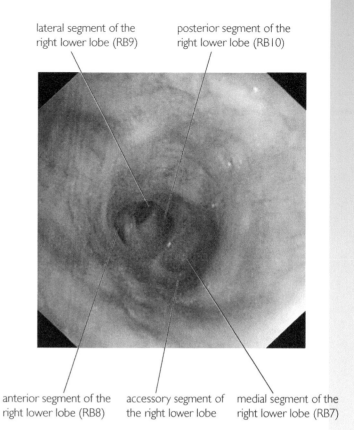

anterior segment of the right lower lobe (RB8)

accessory segment of the right lower lobe

medial segment of the right lower lobe (RB7)

Fig. 3.8p *Endoscopic view of the right lower lobe variant with submedial segment.*

lateral segment of the right lower lobe (RB9)

posterior segment of the right lower lobe (RB10)

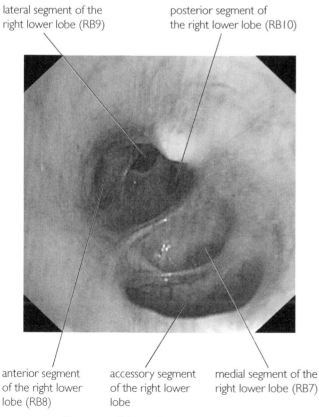

anterior segment of the right lower lobe (RB8)

accessory segment of the right lower lobe

medial segment of the right lower lobe (RB7)

Fig. 3.8q *Close-up of the right lower lobe variant with a submedial segment.*

Left main bronchus (Fig. 3.9)

The left main bronchus is approximately 4 cm long and descends in a gentle lateral curve. At its terminal portion it divides into two main branches: the left lower lobe and the left upper lobe bronchus. There is an obliquely placed sharp carina separating the two bronchi. The upper lobe is joined at a 60° angle to the left main bronchus. Occasionally the upper lobe bronchus joins the left main bronchus at an acute angle.

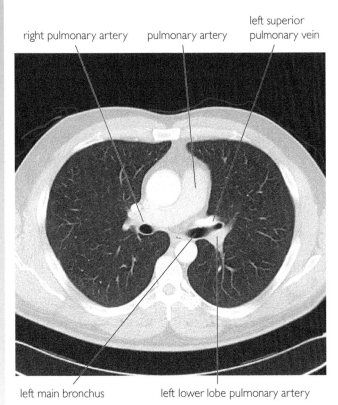

left main bronchus

right pulmonary artery   pulmonary artery   left superior pulmonary vein

left main bronchus   left lower lobe pulmonary artery

Fig. 3.9a *Cross-sectional CT scan of the thorax at the level of the left main bronchus.*

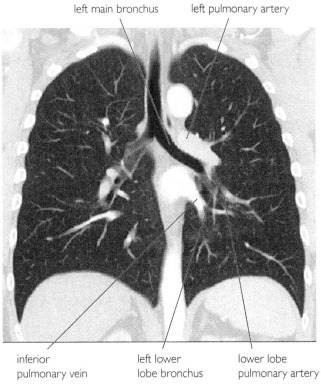

left main bronchus   left pulmonary artery

inferior pulmonary vein   left lower lobe bronchus   lower lobe pulmonary artery

Fig. 3.9b *Coronal sectional CT scan of the thorax at the level of the left main bronchus.*

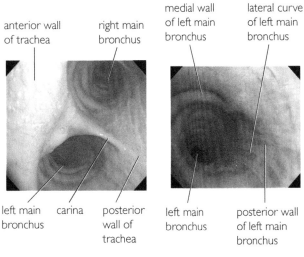

anterior wall of trachea   right main bronchus   medial wall of left main bronchus   lateral curve of left main bronchus

left main bronchus   carina   posterior wall of trachea   left main bronchus   posterior wall of left main bronchus

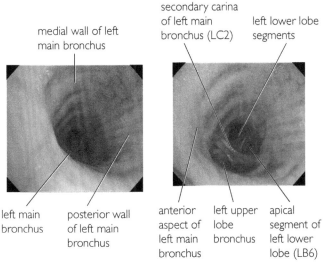

medial wall of left main bronchus   secondary carina of left main bronchus (LC2)   left lower lobe segments

left main bronchus   posterior wall of left main bronchus   anterior aspect of left main bronchus   left upper lobe bronchus   apical segment of left lower lobe (LB6)

Fig. 3.9c *Endoscopic view of the left main bronchus from the carina.*

Fig. 3.9d *Endoscopic view of the curve in the left main bronchus.*

Fig. 3.9e *Endoscopic view of the left main bronchus viewed from halfway down the left main bronchus with the left lower lobe visible distally.*

Fig. 3.9f *Endoscopic view of the left main bronchus viewed from two-thirds the way down the left main bronchus, with the left lower lobe visible distally.*

secondary carina of left main bronchus (LC2)   basal segments of left lower lobe

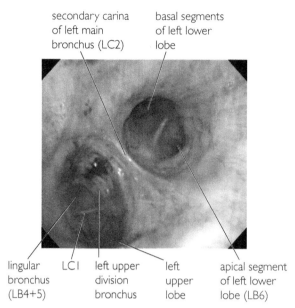

lingular bronchus (LB4+5)   LC1   left upper division bronchus   left upper lobe   apical segment of left lower lobe (LB6)

Fig. 3.9g *Endoscopic view of the left secondary carina with both the upper and lower lobes visible.*

left lower lobe   medial wall of left main bronchus

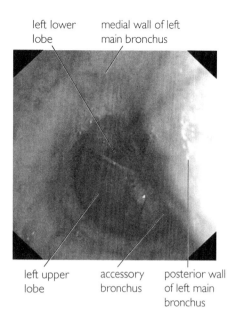

left upper lobe   accessory bronchus   posterior wall of left main bronchus

Fig. 3.9h *Endoscopic view of the left lower and upper lobes, with the apical segment of the left upper lobe arising from the left main bronchus.*

secondary carina   left lower lobe

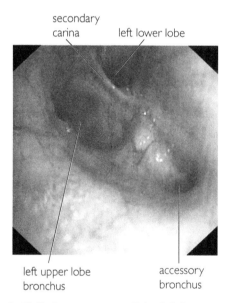

left upper lobe bronchus   accessory bronchus

Fig. 3.9i *Endoscopic view of the left lower and upper lobes with a close view of the apical segment of the left upper lobe arising from the left main bronchus.*

secondary carina   left lower lobe

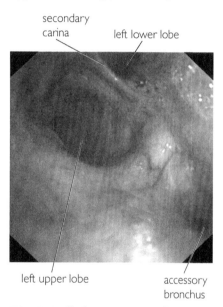

left upper lobe   accessory bronchus

Fig. 3.9j *Endoscopic view of the left lower and upper lobes with a view of the apical segment of the left upper lobe arising from the left main bronchus, just from above its origin.*

Left upper lobe (Fig. 3.10)

The upper lobe bronchus usually divides into the upper division orifice and the lingular bronchus. The upper division divides into an apicoposterior and anterior bronchus. In the majority of individuals, the apicoposterior bronchus divides into three segmental branches: the apical, posterior and posterolateral branches. In about 15 per cent of individuals the apicoposterior segment has a bipartite structure with the posterolateral subsegment arising from the anterior segment.

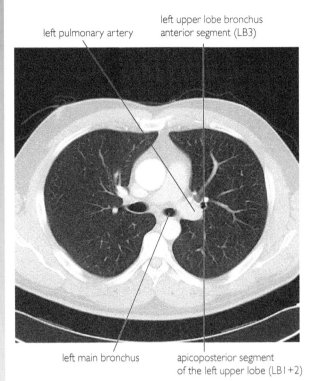

left pulmonary artery

left upper lobe bronchus
anterior segment (LB3)

left main bronchus

apicoposterior segment
of the left upper lobe (LB1+2)

Fig. 3.10a *Cross-sectional CT scan of the thorax at the level of the left upper lobe bronchus.*

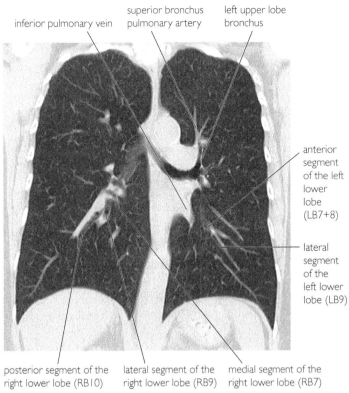

inferior pulmonary vein

superior bronchus
pulmonary artery

left upper lobe
bronchus

anterior segment of the left lower lobe (LB7+8)

lateral segment of the left lower lobe (LB9)

posterior segment of the right lower lobe (RB10)

lateral segment of the right lower lobe (RB9)

medial segment of the right lower lobe (RB7)

Fig. 3.10b *Coronal sectional CT scan of the thorax at the level of the left upper lobe bronchus.*

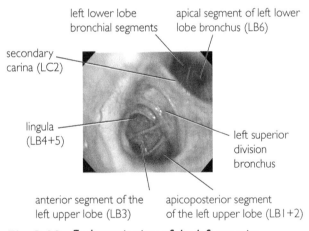

left lower lobe bronchial segments

apical segment of left lower lobe bronchus (LB6)

secondary carina (LC2)

lingula (LB4+5)

left superior division bronchus

anterior segment of the left upper lobe (LB3)

apicoposterior segment of the left upper lobe (LB1+2)

Fig. 3.10c *Endoscopic view of the left superior bronchus from above the left main bronchial carina.*

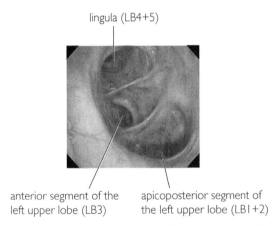

lingula (LB4+5)

anterior segment of the left upper lobe (LB3)

apicoposterior segment of the left upper lobe (LB1+2)

Fig. 3.10d *Close-up of the left superior bronchus showing the lingula and left upper lobe segments.*

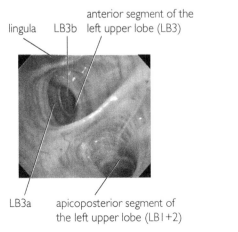

lingula   LB3b   anterior segment of the left upper lobe (LB3)

LB3a   apicoposterior segment of the left upper lobe (LB1+2)

Fig. 3.10e *Left upper lobe segments showing anterior and apicoposterior segments.*

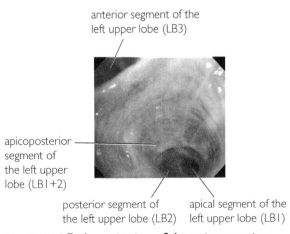

anterior segment of the left upper lobe (LB3)

apicoposterior segment of the left upper lobe (LB1+2)

posterior segment of the left upper lobe (LB2)

apical segment of the left upper lobe (LB1)

Fig. 3.10f *Endoscopic view of the apicoposterior segment of the left upper lobe.*

Lingula (Fig. 3.11)

The lingular bronchus arises from the left upper division bronchus. It divides into superior segmental and inferior segmental branches, which in turn divide into two subsegmental branches. In 25 per cent of individuals, the lingula bifurcates in a lateral and medial fashion. On rare occasions the orifice of the lingula is merged with a segment from the upper lobe.

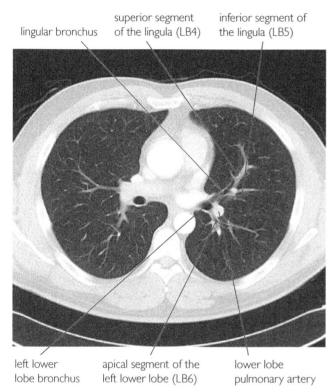

superior segment of the lingula (LB4)

inferior segment of the lingula (LB5)

lingular bronchus

left lower lobe bronchus

apical segment of the left lower lobe (LB6)

lower lobe pulmonary artery

Fig. 3.11a *Cross-sectional CT scan of the thorax at the level of the lingular bronchus.*

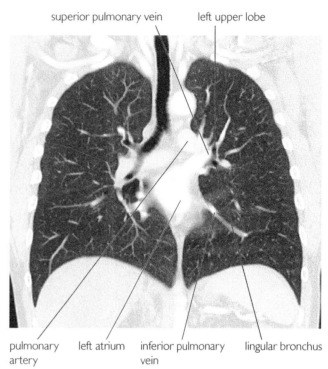

superior pulmonary vein

left upper lobe

pulmonary artery

left atrium

inferior pulmonary vein

lingular bronchus

Fig. 3.11b *Coronal sectional CT scan of the thorax at the level of the lingular bronchus.*

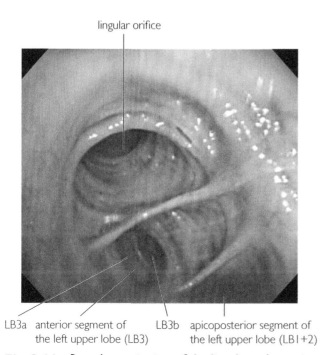

lingular orifice

LB3a anterior segment of the left upper lobe (LB3)

LB3b apicoposterior segment of the left upper lobe (LB1+2)

Fig. 3.11c *Bronchoscopic view of the lingula and anterior segment of the left upper lobe.*

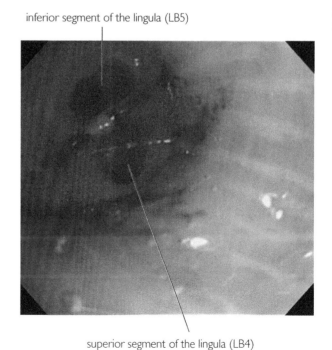

inferior segment of the lingula (LB5)

superior segment of the lingula (LB4)

Fig. 3.11d *Endoscopic view of the lingular segments.*

Left lower lobe (Fig. 3.12)

The left lower lobe bronchus descends posterolaterally and divides into four segments to form the left lower lobe. The apical segment arises about 1 cm after the origin of the left lower lobe bronchus. After a further 1–2 cm the inferior bronchus divides into an anterior basal segmental bronchus and a posterolateral basal bronchus which further bifurcates into lateral basal and posterior basal segments. Endoscopically a prominent secondary carina appears to divide into the apical basal bronchus and the other inferior branches. The most common pattern of division of the left lower lobe is into three branches (tripartite) with separate anterior basal, lateral basal and posterior basal divisions.

superior segment of the lingula (LB4)

left pulmonary artery

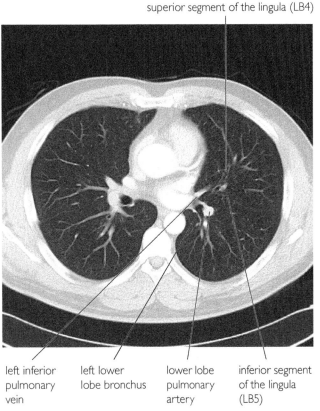 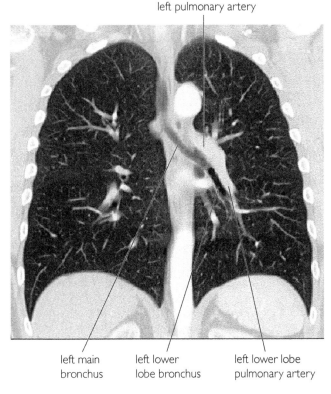

left inferior pulmonary vein

left lower lobe bronchus

lower lobe pulmonary artery

inferior segment of the lingula (LB5)

left main bronchus

left lower lobe bronchus

left lower lobe pulmonary artery

Fig. 3.12a *Cross-sectional CT scan of the thorax at the level of the left lower lobe bronchus.*

Fig. 3.12b *Coronal sectional CT scan of the thorax at the level of the left lower lobe bronchus.*

basal segments of the left lower lobe

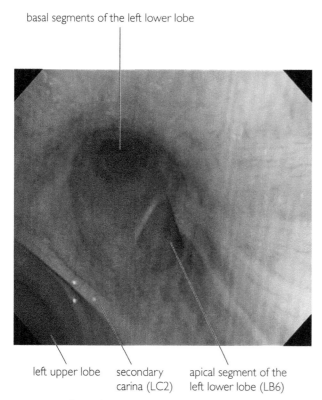

left upper lobe   secondary carina (LC2)   apical segment of the left lower lobe (LB6)

Fig. 3.12c *Bronchoscopic view of the left lower lobe viewed from just above the left secondary carina.*

basal segments of the left lower lobe

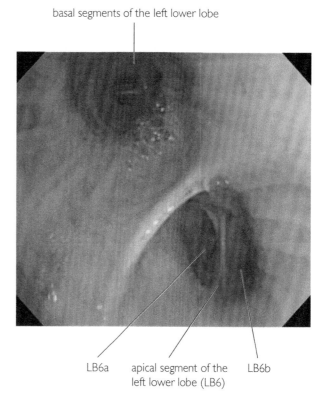

LB6a   apical segment of the left lower lobe (LB6)   LB6b

Fig. 3.12d *Endoscopic view of the left lower lobe.*

basal segments of the left lower lobe

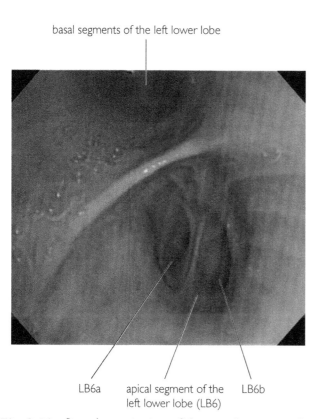

LB6a   apical segment of the left lower lobe (LB6)   LB6b

Fig. 3.12e *Bronchoscopic view of the apical segment of the left lower lobe.*

lateral segment of the left lower lobe (LB9)   posterior segment of the left lower lobe (LB10)

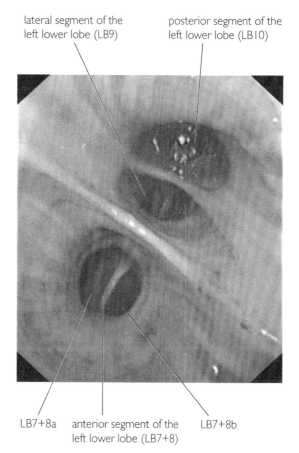

LB7+8a   anterior segment of the left lower lobe (LB7+8)   LB7+8b

Fig. 3.12f *Bronchoscopic view of the basal segments of the left lower lobe.*

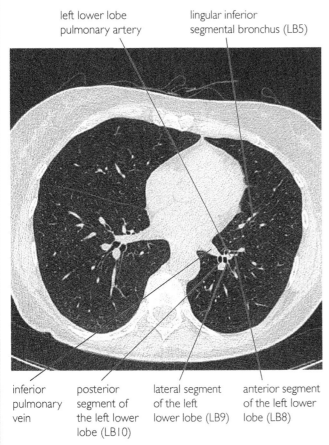

left lower lobe
pulmonary artery

lingular inferior
segmental bronchus (LB5)

inferior
pulmonary
vein

posterior
segment of
the left lower
lobe (LB10)

lateral segment
of the left
lower lobe (LB9)

anterior segment
of the left lower
lobe (LB8)

Fig. 3.12g *Cross-sectional CT scan of the thorax showing the left lower lobe segments.*

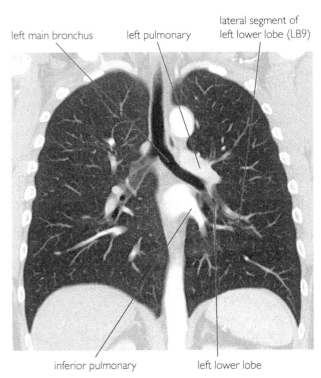

left main bronchus

left pulmonary

lateral segment of
left lower lobe (LB9)

inferior pulmonary

left lower lobe

Fig. 3.12h *Coronal sectional CT scan of the thorax showing the left lower lobe segments.*

Normal anatomy (posterior approach)

In this chapter the endoscopic images are related to the computed tomography (CT) images. The overall appearance, main characteristics and normal variations are described. Here, in contrast to Chapter 3, the endoscopic images are presented as they appear when the patient is bronchoscoped in a supine position and approached from behind.

Vocal cords (Fig. 4.1)

The larynx is composed of a series of cartilages, ligaments and fibrous membranes. At bronchoscopy the epiglottis is the more proximal structure. It is a broad leaf-like structure. The sides are attached by the arytenoid cartilages. The cuneiform and corniculate can be seen at the end of the arytenoid cartilage. The cuneiform cartilage is more anterior and superior to the corniculate cartilage. The vocal folds consist of the false cords or vestibular folds and the true vocal folds. They stretch back from the thyroid angle to the vocal processes of the arytenoids. The vocal folds are involved in the production of sound.

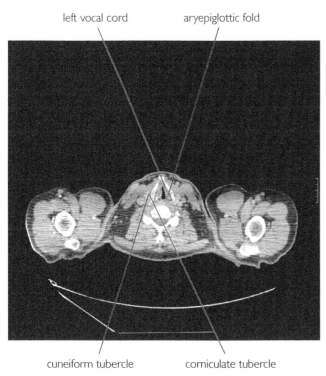

Fig. 4.1a *Cross-sectional CT scan at the superior aspect of the thorax at the level of the vocal cords, which are apposed.*

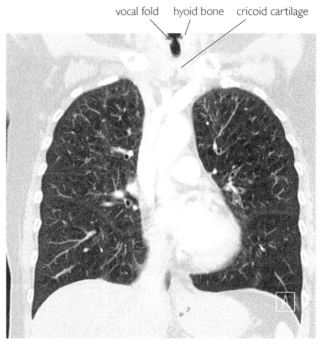

Fig. 4.1b *Coronal section CT scan of the vocal cords, which are apposed.*

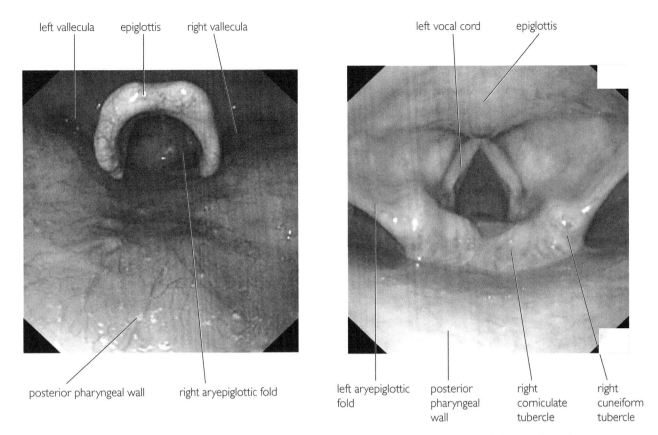

left vallecula   epiglottis   right vallecula

posterior pharyngeal wall   right aryepiglottic fold

Fig. 4.1c *Endoscopic view of the epiglottis and vocal cords.*

left vocal cord   epiglottis

left aryepiglottic fold   posterior pharyngeal wall   right corniculate tubercle   right cuneiform tubercle

Fig. 4.1d *Endoscopic view of the vocal cords.*

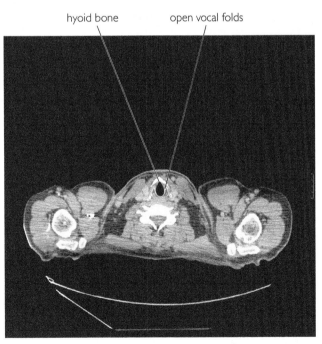

hyoid bone   open vocal folds

Fig. 4.1e *Cross-sectional CT scan at the superior aspect of the thorax at the level of the vocal cords, which are open.*

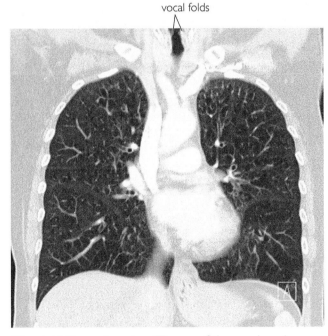

vocal folds

Fig. 4.1f *Coronal section CT scan of the vocal cords, which are open.*

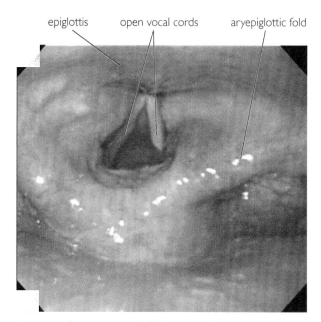

epiglottis   open vocal cords   aryepiglottic fold

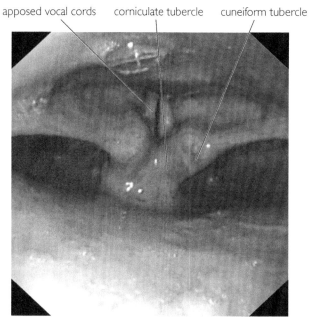

apposed vocal cords   corniculate tubercle   cuneiform tubercle

Fig. 4.1g *Cross-sectional CT scan at the superior aspect of the thorax at the level of the vocal cords.*

Fig. 4.1h *Coronal section CT of the vocal cords, which are apposed.*

Trachea (Fig. 4.2)

The trachea is a horseshoe- or D-shaped structure which extends from the cricoid cartilage to the carina. The anterior aspect is composed of 16–20 incomplete cartilage rings with a flat fibromuscular posterior component. There is also a longitudinal band of connective tissue which runs down the posterior end of the cartilage. At bronchoscopy the cartilage bands on the anterior surface appear as ridges and the posterior wall appears to bulge into the trachea. The posterior bulge is accentuated in expiration.

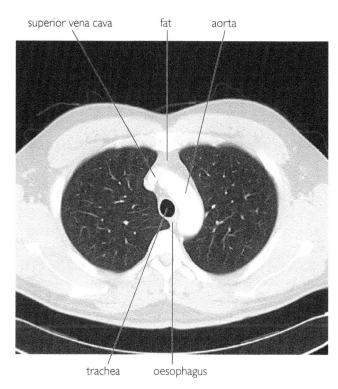

superior vena cava   fat   aorta

trachea   oesophagus

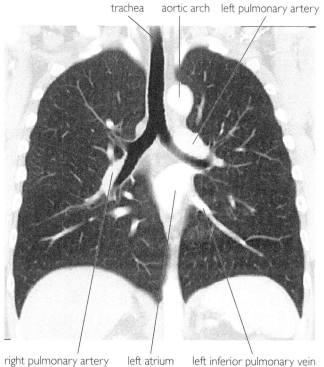

trachea   aortic arch   left pulmonary artery

right pulmonary artery   left atrium   left inferior pulmonary vein

Fig. 4.2a *Cross-sectional CT scan of the thorax at the mid-tracheal level.*

Fig. 4.2b *Coronal sectional CT scan of the thorax through the trachea.*

cartilage rings   anterior aspect

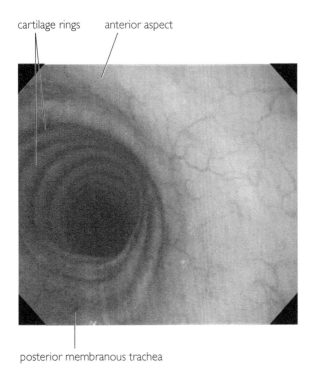

posterior membranous trachea

Fig. 4.2c *Endoscopic view of the trachea from the level of the subglottis.*

carina   anterior wall   cartilage rings

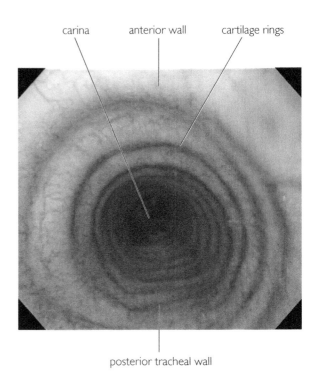

posterior tracheal wall

Fig. 4.2d *Endoscopic view of the upper trachea.*

anterior
tracheal   left main   right main
wall   bronchus   bronchus

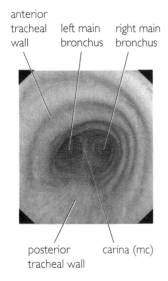

posterior   carina (mc)
tracheal wall

Fig. 4.2e *Endoscopic view of the trachea from the mid-tracheal level.*

left main   anterior   right main
bronchus   aspect   bronchus

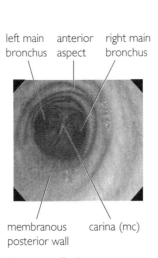

membranous   carina (mc)
posterior wall

Fig. 4.2f *Endoscopic view of the distal portion of the trachea.*

anterior   right
aspect of   upper   tracheal
trachea   lobe   bronchus

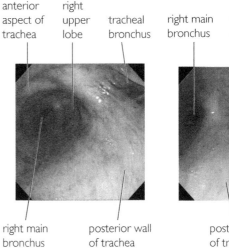

right main   posterior wall
bronchus   of trachea

Fig. 4.2g *Endoscopic view of a tracheal bronchus as viewed from above with the patient supine and approached from behind. The right upper lobe arises from the right main bronchus.*

right
right   upper   tracheal
right main   upper   tracheal
bronchus   lobe   bronchus

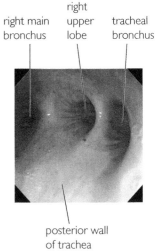

posterior wall
of trachea

Fig. 4.2h *Endoscopic view of a tracheal bronchus as seen at the distal trachea just above the carina. The right upper lobe and bronchus intermedius are visible below.*

anterior segment of the right upper lobe

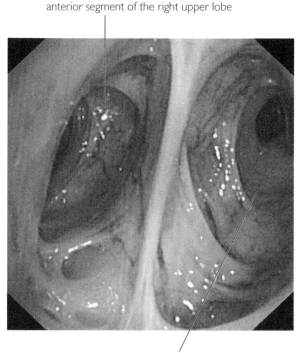

posterior segment of the right upper lobe

Fig. 4.2i *Bipartite division of the upper lobe in the presence of a tracheal bronchus.*

tracheal bronchus   trachea

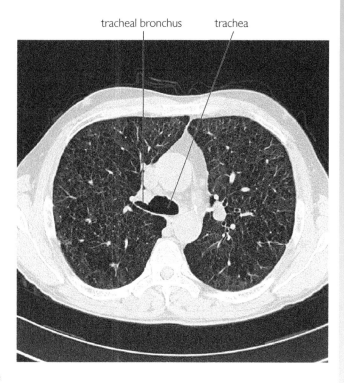

Fig. 4.2j *Cross-sectional CT scan showing the tracheal bronchus arising at the distal trachea just above the carina.*

The trachea measures approximately 110 mm in length with an external diameter that ranges from 15 mm in women to 20 mm in men. The internal diameter of the trachea is about 12–14 mm.

The trachea divides into the right and left main bronchi at the level of the sternomanubrial junction or the body of the fourth thoracic vertebrae.

A tracheal bronchus is a rare normal variant and originates from the lateral wall of the trachea and into the upper lobe on the right side in about 0.1–2 per cent of individuals and on the left side in 0.3–1 per cent of individuals. The term tracheal bronchus is also used for other anomalous airways arising from the main bronchi and directed to the upper lobes.

Carina (Fig. 4.3)

The carina is a concave spur of cartilage located where the distal trachea divides into the right and left main bronchi. The carina normally appears as a sharp structure and forms the medial borders of the origin of the right and left main bronchi. The sharp angle is maintained as it is primarily composed of cartilage (carinal) and ligaments (interbronchial). Enlargement of the subcarinal structures, such as the subcarinal lymph nodes or the left atrium, may lead to blunting or widening of the carina. It usually measures about 12 mm in diameter and stretches in the midline in the anteroposterior dimension. Very rarely there is an accessory bronchus opening from the lateral walls directed towards the upper lobe.

apical segment of the right upper lobe (RB1)   superior vena cava   ascending aorta   pulmonary artery   anterior segment of the left upper lobe (LB3)   oblique fissure

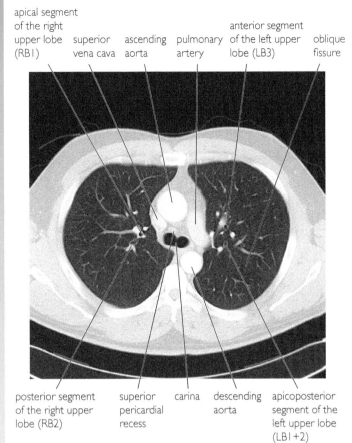

posterior segment of the right upper lobe (RB2)   superior pericardial recess   carina   descending aorta   apicoposterior segment of the left upper lobe (LB1+2)

Fig. 4.3a *Cross-sectional CT scan of the thorax at the level of the carina.*

right pulmonary artery   right upper lobe   apicoposterior segment of the left upper lobe (LB1+2)

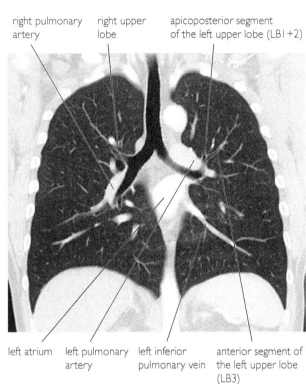

left atrium   left pulmonary artery   left inferior pulmonary vein   anterior segment of the left upper lobe (LB3)

Fig. 4.3b *Coronal sectional CT scan of the thorax through the trachea.*

left main bronchus   carina (mc)   right main bronchus

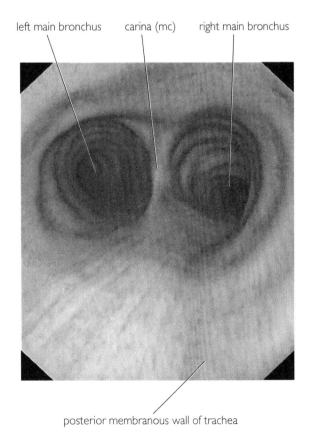

posterior membranous wall of trachea

Fig. 4.3c *Endoscopic view of the carina.*

left main bronchus   carina (mc)   right main bronchus

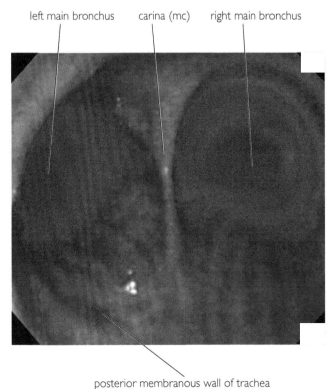

posterior membranous wall of trachea

Fig. 4.3d *Close-up endoscopic view of the carina.*

Right main bronchus (Fig. 4.4)

The right main bronchus extends from the carina to the origin of the right upper lobe. It then forms the bronchus intermedius. The right main bronchus has a steeper decline from the trachea and hence, in the upright position, foreign bodies tend to fall into the right main bronchus. It is slightly larger in diameter than the left main bronchus, measuring between 10 and 12 mm in external diameter. The inferior lip of the upper lobe bronchus is easily visible at the distal end of the right main bronchus. A rare variation is the origin of an airway leading to the upper lobe. This is classified as a pre-eparterial tracheal bronchus. It may be either a supernumerary or a displaced airway. Where the airway is displaced, there is also a missing upper lobe branch. An accessory cardiac bronchus is a supernumerary bronchus arising from the medial aspect of the right main bronchus and leading towards the pericardium.

anterior segmental bronchus of right upper lobe (RB3) apical segmental bronchus of right upper lobe (RB1) superior vena cava carina (mc)

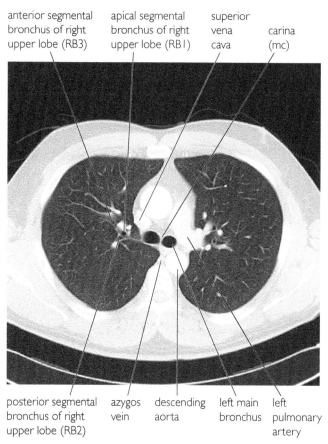

posterior segmental bronchus of right upper lobe (RB2) azygos vein descending aorta left main bronchus left pulmonary artery

Fig. 4.4a *Cross-sectional CT scan of the thorax at the carina, showing the right main lobe.*

azygos arch trachea carina (mc) left main bronchus

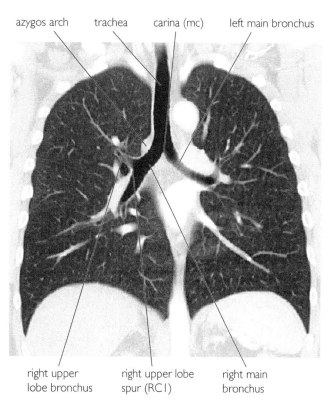

right upper lobe bronchus right upper lobe spur (RC1) right main bronchus

Fig. 4.4b *Coronal sectional CT scan of the thorax showing the right main bronchus.*

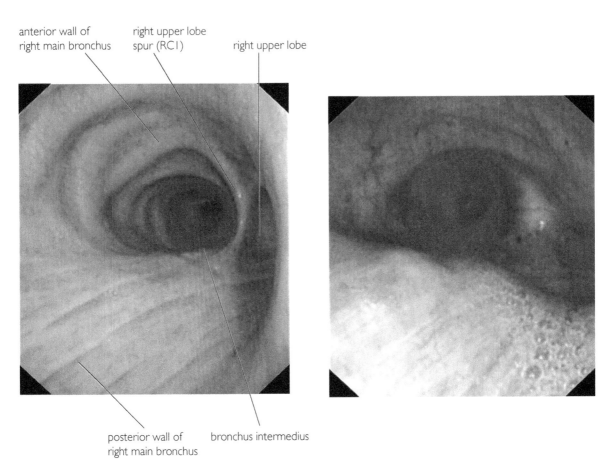

anterior wall of
right main bronchus

right upper lobe
spur (RC1)

right upper lobe

posterior wall of
right main bronchus

bronchus intermedius

Fig. 4.4c *Endoscopic view of the right main bronchus visible below the carina.*

Fig. 4.4d *Endoscopic view of the right main bronchus which shows more of the right upper lobe origin.*

Right upper lobe (Fig. 4.5)

The right upper lobe has three main segmental divisions: the apical, anterior and posterior segments. The upper lobe segments divide into segments about 10 mm from the origin. The upper lobe is subject to considerable normal variation:

- In 40 per cent the segmental bronchi arise independently.
- In 24 per cent there is a common apical and anterior trunk and an independent post-segmental bronchus. (See Fig 4.5g)
- In 14 per cent there is a common apical and posterior trunk and an independent anterior segment. (See Fig 4.5h)
- In 10 per cent there is a common anterior and posterior trunk with an independent apical segment.
- In 10 per cent the posterior segmental bronchus is absent.
- In 2 per cent the apical segment is absent.
- In < 1 per cent of patients there is a tracheal bronchus which originates either directly from the trachea or at the level of the carina. In some cases there is an additional branch to the upper lobe, which originates from the right main bronchus.

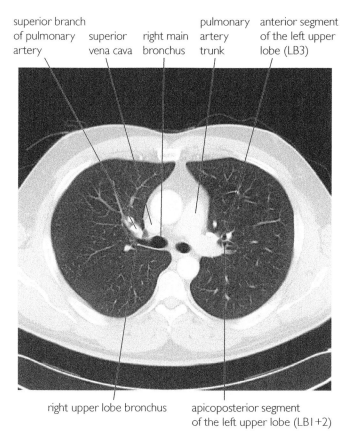

superior branch of pulmonary artery | superior vena cava | right main bronchus | pulmonary artery trunk | anterior segment of the left upper lobe (LB3)

right upper lobe bronchus | apicoposterior segment of the left upper lobe (LB1+2)

Fig. 4.5a *Cross-sectional CT scan of the thorax at the level of the right upper lobe origin.*

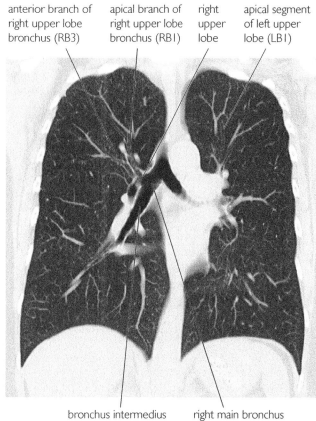

anterior branch of right upper lobe bronchus (RB3) | apical branch of right upper lobe bronchus (RB1) | right upper lobe | apical segment of left upper lobe (LB1)

bronchus intermedius | right main bronchus

Fig. 4.5b *Coronal sectional CT scan of the thorax showing the right upper lobe.*

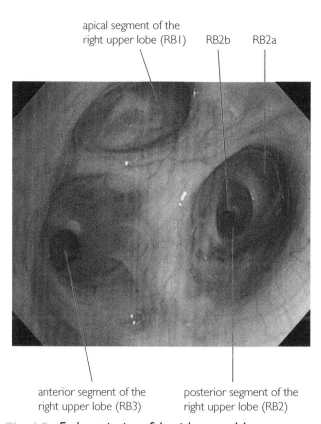

apical segment of the right upper lobe (RB1) | RB2b | RB2a

anterior segment of the right upper lobe (RB3) | posterior segment of the right upper lobe (RB2)

Fig. 4.5c *Endoscopic view of the right upper lobe.*

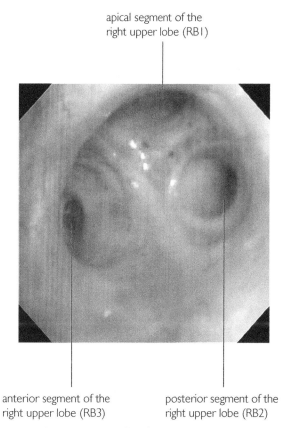

apical segment of the right upper lobe (RB1)

anterior segment of the right upper lobe (RB3) | posterior segment of the right upper lobe (RB2)

Fig. 4.5d *Another example of the tripartite right upper lobe arrangement.*

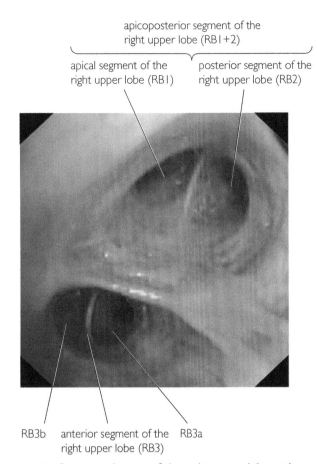

apicoposterior segment of the
right upper lobe (RB1+2)

apical segment of the
right upper lobe (RB1)

posterior segment of the
right upper lobe (RB2)

RB3b   anterior segment of the   RB3a
          right upper lobe (RB3)

Fig. 4.5e *Bipartite division of the right upper lobe with division at the horizontal axis.*

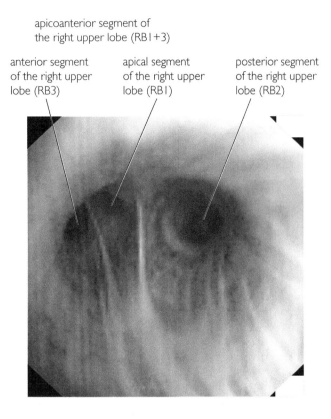

apicoanterior segment of
the right upper lobe (RB1+3)

anterior segment
of the right upper
lobe (RB3)

apical segment
of the right upper
lobe (RB1)

posterior segment
of the right upper
lobe (RB2)

Fig. 4.5f *Bipartite division of the right upper lobe with division in the vertical axis.*

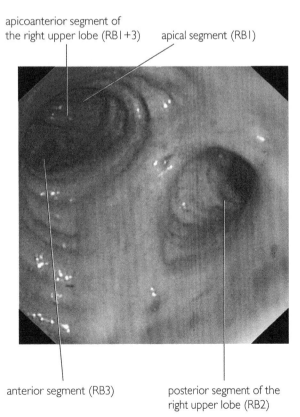

apicoanterior segment of
the right upper lobe (RB1+3)

apical segment (RB1)

anterior segment (RB3)

posterior segment of the
right upper lobe (RB2)

Fig. 4.5g *Bipartite division of the right upper lobe with apical and anterior segments (RB1 + 3 arising together) and a separate posterior segment (RB2).*

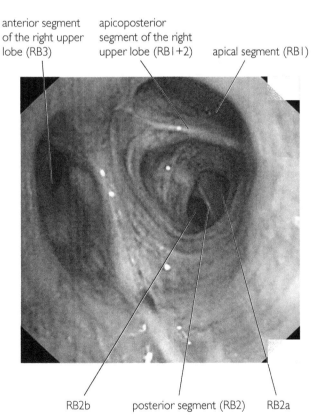

anterior segment
of the right upper
lobe (RB3)

apicoposterior
segment of the right
upper lobe (RB1+2)

apical segment (RB1)

RB2b   posterior segment (RB2)   RB2a

Fig. 4.5h *Bipartite division of the right upper lobe with apical and posterior segments arising together (RB1 + 2) and a separate posterior segment (RB3).*

anterior segment of the right upper lobe (RB3)

apical segment of the right upper lobe (RB1)

apicoposterior segment of the right upper lobe (RB1+2)

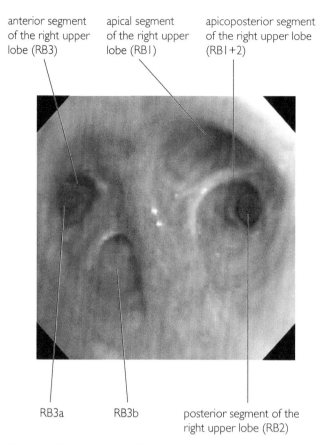

RB3a

RB3b

posterior segment of the right upper lobe (RB2)

Fig. 4.5i *Four divisions of the right upper lobe.*

Bronchus intermedius (Fig. 4.6)

The bronchus intermedius originates from the right main bronchus and extends from the origin of the right upper lobe to the right middle lobe. It is approximately 20 mm long and has a diameter of about 10 mm. The right middle lobe, the apical segment of the lower lobe and the basal segments are visible at the distal end of bronchus intermedius.

bronchus intermedius | left ventricular outflow tract | pulmonary trunk | left main bronchus | left superior pulmonary vein

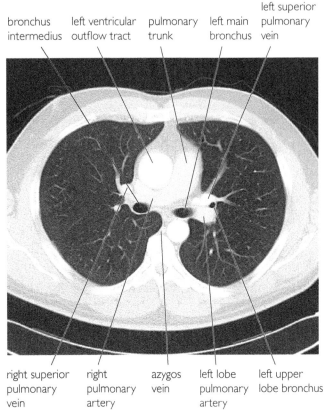

right superior pulmonary vein | right pulmonary artery | azygos vein | left lobe pulmonary artery | left upper lobe bronchus

Fig. 4.6a *Cross-sectional CT scan of the thorax at the level of the bronchus intermedius (distal to the right upper lobe origin).*

right upper lobe bronchus | apicoposterior segment of the left upper lobe (LB1+2) | anterior segment of the left upper lobe (LB3)

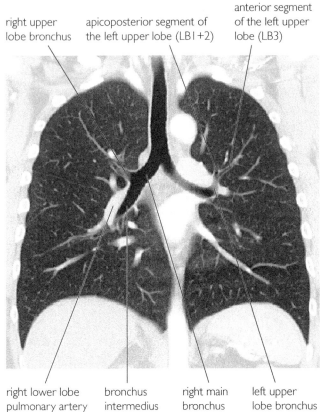

right lower lobe pulmonary artery | bronchus intermedius | right main bronchus | left upper lobe bronchus

Fig. 4.6b *Coronal sectional CT scan of the thorax through the bronchial tree showing the bronchus intermedius.*

right middle lobe (RB4+5)

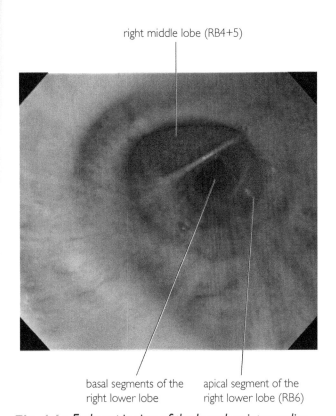

basal segments of the right lower lobe | apical segment of the right lower lobe (RB6)

Fig. 4.6c *Endoscopic view of the bronchus intermedius.*

right middle lobe bronchus (RB4+5) | carina between right middle lobe and lower lobe (RC2)

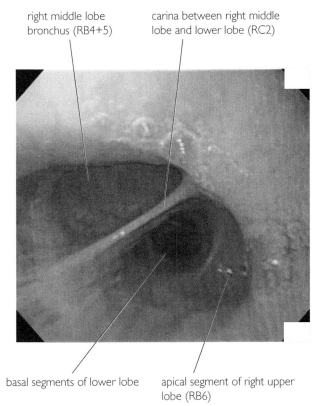

basal segments of lower lobe | apical segment of right upper lobe (RB6)

Fig. 4.6d *Endoscopic view of the distal aspect of the bronchus intermedius.*

Right middle lobe (Fig. 4.7)

The right middle lobe is a semi-lunar (D-shaped) bronchus at the anterior end of the bronchus intermedius. In approximately 70 per cent of cases, there are two distinct segments: lateral and medial. In 23 per cent of normal individuals the middle lobe bifurcates in a superior-inferior fashion, similar to that of the lingula. In up to 20 per cent of individuals there is a main lateral bronchus and a smaller medial bronchus which arises from the lateral segment. Occasionally the reverse is seen, with a larger medial segment and a smaller lateral segment arising from it.

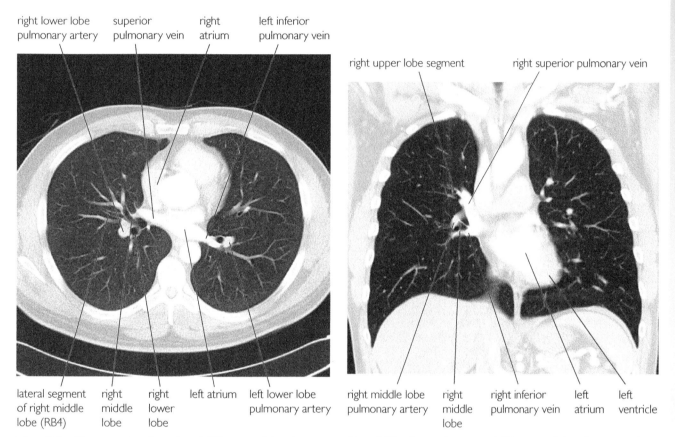

Fig. 4.7a *Cross-sectional sectional CT scan of the thorax at the level of the right middle lobe.*

Fig. 4.7b *Coronal sectional CT scan of the thorax at the level of the right middle lobe.*

right middle lobe

carina between right middle
lobe and lower lobe (RC2)

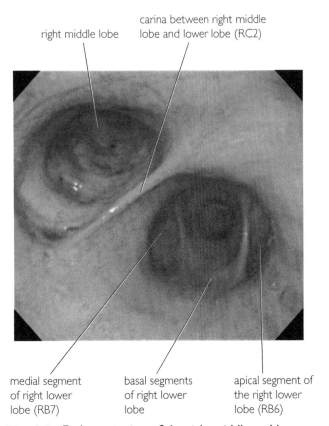

medial segment
of right lower
lobe (RB7)

basal segments
of right lower
lobe

apical segment of
the right lower
lobe (RB6)

Fig. 4.7c *Endoscopic view of the right middle and lower lobes.*

right middle lobe

carina between right middle lobe
and right lower lobe (RC2)

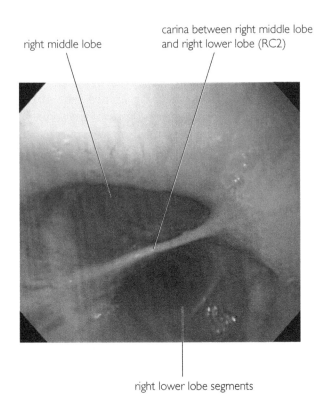

right lower lobe segments

Fig. 4.7d *Endoscopic view of the right middle lobe.*

RB5b   RB5a

medial segment of the
right lower lobe (RB5)

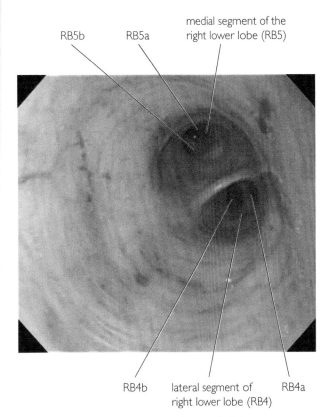

RB4b

lateral segment of
right lower lobe (RB4)

RB4a

Fig. 4.7e *Endoscopic view of right middle lobe subsegments viewed from the origin of the right main bronchus.*

medial segment of the
right middle lobe (RB5)

RB5b   RB5a

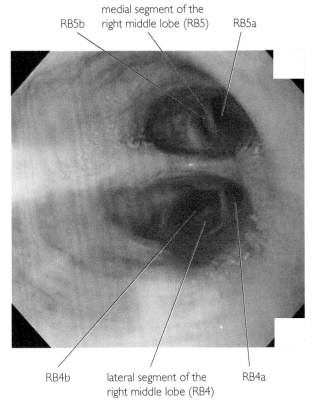

RB4b

lateral segment of the
right middle lobe (RB4)

RB4a

Fig. 4.7f *Close-up endoscopic view of the right middle lobe subsegments.*

Right lower lobe (Fig. 4.8)

The right lower lobe comprises five main segments: apical basal, medial basal, anterior basal, lateral basal and posterior basal. In about 40–60 per cent of individuals there is an additional subapical basal segment. The apical basal segment of the right lower lobe is positioned posteriorly at the end of the bronchus intermedius. The apical segment divides immediately into three subsegmental bronchi. The normal pattern observed in the lower lobe bronchial segments are a large medial basal segment (RB7), which is proximal to the other basal segments. The anterior basal segment is in the lateral position, with the lower bronchus dividing further into lateral and posterior segments. This pattern is seen in over 70 per cent of individuals. The other common variation observed is where the anterior basal, lateral basal and posterior basal segments all originate independently at the same level.

A bipartite division is occasionally observed where the anterior and lateral segments arise together proximally to the posterior basal segment from a separate branch. The position and size of the apical basal segment frequently influence the pattern of branching of the basal segments. For example, in some individuals there is a larger apical bronchus and, as a result, the medial through to posterior segment arises in a tripartite from the same level.

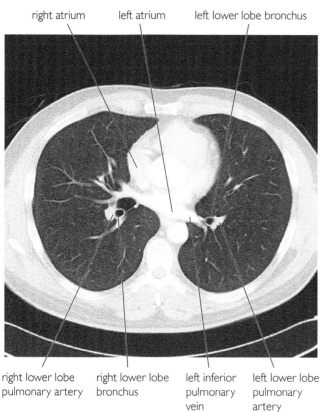

right atrium   left atrium   left lower lobe bronchus

right lower lobe pulmonary artery   right lower lobe bronchus   left inferior pulmonary vein   left lower lobe pulmonary artery

Fig. 4.8a *Cross-sectional CT scan of the thorax at the level of the right lower lobe.*

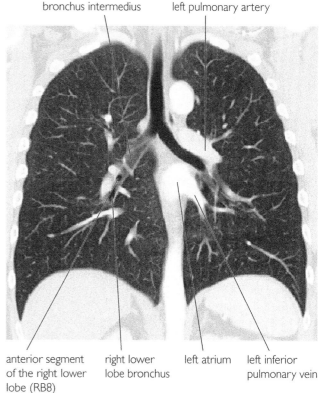

bronchus intermedius   left pulmonary artery

anterior segment of the right lower lobe (RB8)   right lower lobe bronchus   left atrium   left inferior pulmonary vein

Fig. 4.8b *Coronal sectional CT scan showing the right lower lobe.*

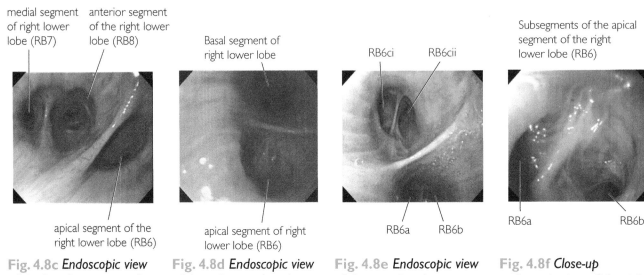

medial segment of right lower lobe (RB7)

anterior segment of the right lower lobe (RB8)

apical segment of the right lower lobe (RB6)

Basal segment of right lower lobe

apical segment of right lower lobe (RB6)

RB6ci   RB6cii

RB6a   RB6b

Subsegments of the apical segment of the right lower lobe (RB6)

RB6a   RB6b

Fig. 4.8c *Endoscopic view of the basal segments of the right lower lobe.*

Fig. 4.8d *Endoscopic view of the right apicobasal segment.*

Fig. 4.8e *Endoscopic view of the apicobasal segments of the right lower lobe.*

Fig. 4.8f *Close-up endoscopic view of the right apicobasal subsegments.*

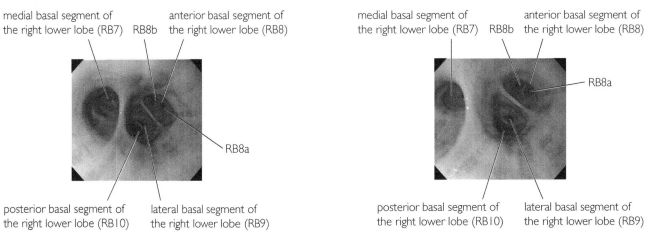

medial basal segment of the right lower lobe (RB7)   RB8b

anterior basal segment of the right lower lobe (RB8)

RB8a

posterior basal segment of the right lower lobe (RB10)

lateral basal segment of the right lower lobe (RB9)

medial basal segment of the right lower lobe (RB7)   RB8b

anterior basal segment of the right lower lobe (RB8)

RB8a

posterior basal segment of the right lower lobe (RB10)

lateral basal segment of the right lower lobe (RB9)

Fig. 4.8g *Endoscopic view of the basal segments of the right lower lobe.*

Fig. 4.8h *Closer endoscopic view of the basal segments of the right lower lobe.*

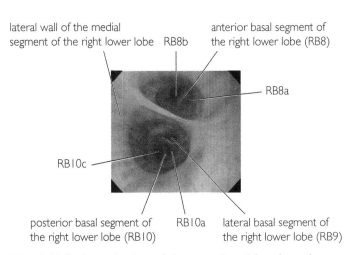

lateral wall of the medial segment of the right lower lobe   RB8b

anterior basal segment of the right lower lobe (RB8)

RB8a

RB10c

posterior basal segment of the right lower lobe (RB10)

RB10a

lateral basal segment of the right lower lobe (RB9)

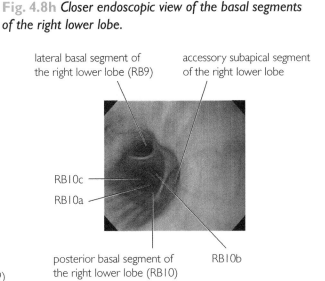

lateral basal segment of the right lower lobe (RB9)

accessory subapical segment of the right lower lobe

RB10c
RB10a

posterior basal segment of the right lower lobe (RB10)

RB10b

Fig. 4.8i *Endoscopic view of the anterobasal, basolateral and posterobasal segments of the right lower lobe.*

Fig. 4.8j *Endoscopic view of the basolateral and posterobasal segments of the right lower lobe. In this example a normal variant subapical segment is present.*

anterior segment right lower lobe (RB8)

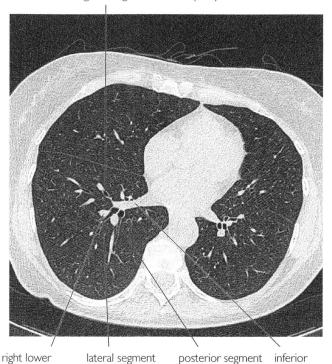

right lower lobe pulmonary artery

lateral segment of the right lower lobe (RB9)

posterior segment of right lower lobe (RB10)

inferior pulmonary vein

Fig. 4.8k *Cross sectional Ct scan at the level of the basal segments of the right lower lobe.*

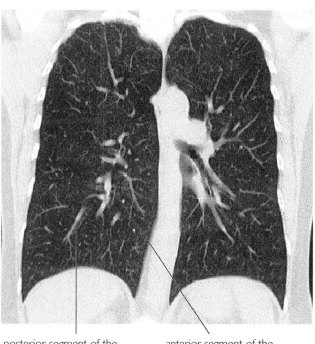

posterior segment of the right lower lobe (RB10)

anterior segment of the right lower lobe (RB8)

Fig. 4.8l *Coronal Ct scan showing the basal segments of the right lower lobe.*

posterior segment of the right lower lobe (RB10)

anterior basal segment of the right lower lobe (RB8)

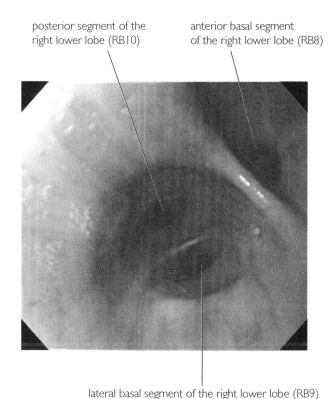

lateral basal segment of the right lower lobe (RB9)

Fig. 4.8m *Endoscopic view of the anterobasal, basolateral and posterobasal segments of the right lower lobe.*

lateral segment of the right lower lobe (RB9)

posterior segment of the right lower lobe (RB10)

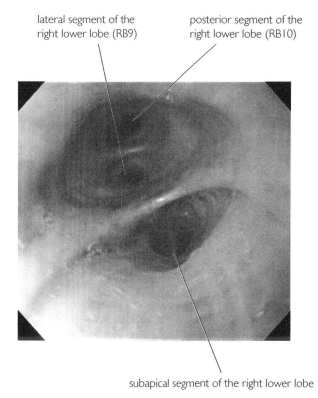

subapical segment of the right lower lobe

Fig. 4.8n *Endoscopic view of the basolateral and posterobasal segments of the right lower lobe.*

medial segment of
the right lower lobe

RB7a

anterior segment of the
right lower lobe (RB8)

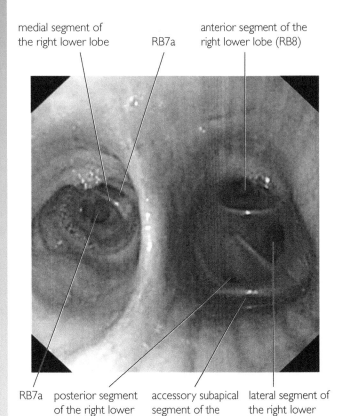

RB7a   posterior segment   accessory subapical   lateral segment of
        of the right lower   segment of the   the right lower
        lobe (RB10)   right lower lobe   lobe (RB9)

Fig. 4.8o *Endoscopic view of the basal segments of the right lower lobe showing a normal variant of a subapical segment.*

medial segment of
the right lower lobe
(RB7)

accessory segment
of the right lower
lobe

anterior segment
of the right lower
lobe (RB8)

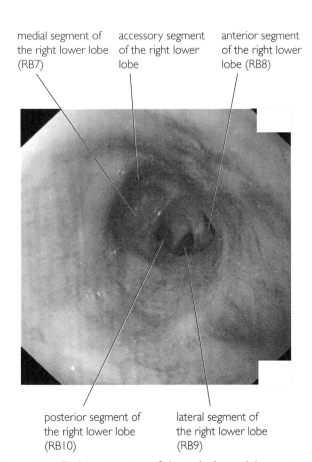

posterior segment of
the right lower lobe
(RB10)

lateral segment of
the right lower lobe
(RB9)

Fig. 4.8p *Endoscopic view of the right lower lobe variant with submedial segment.*

medial segment of the
right lower lobe (RB7)

accessory segment of
the right lower lobe

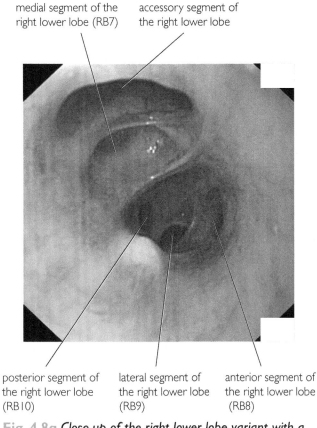

posterior segment of
the right lower lobe
(RB10)

lateral segment of
the right lower lobe
(RB9)

anterior segment of
the right lower lobe
(RB8)

Fig. 4.8q *Close-up of the right lower lobe variant with a submedial segment.*

Left main bronchus (Fig. 4.9)

The left main bronchus is approximately 4 cm long and descends in a gentle lateral curve. At its terminal portion it divides into two main branches: the left lower lobe and the left upper lobe bronchus. There is an obliquely placed sharp carina separating the two bronchi. The upper lobe is joined at a 60° angle to the left main bronchus. Occasionally the upper lobe bronchus joins the left main bronchus at an acute angle.

right pulmonary artery   pulmonary artery   left superior pulmonary vein

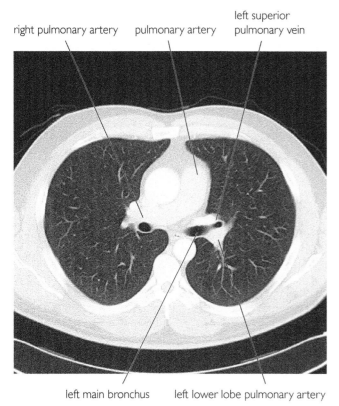

left main bronchus   left lower lobe pulmonary artery

Fig. 4.9a *Cross-sectional CT scan of the thorax at the level of the left main bronchus.*

left main bronchus   left pulmonary artery

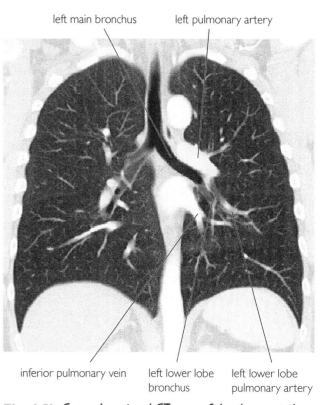

inferior pulmonary vein   left lower lobe bronchus   left lower lobe pulmonary artery

Fig. 4.9b *Coronal sectional CT scan of the thorax at the level of the left main bronchus.*

left main bronchus   anterior wall of trachea

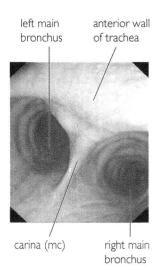

carina (mc)   right main bronchus

Fig. 4.9c *Endoscopic view of the left main bronchus from the carina.*

left main bronchus   medial wall of left main bronchus

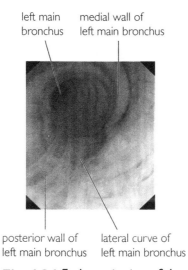

posterior wall of left main bronchus   lateral curve of left main bronchus

Fig. 4.9d *Endoscopic view of the curve in the left main bronchus.*

left main bronchus   medial wall of left main bronchus

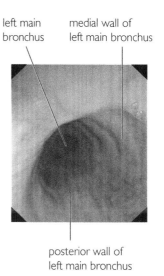

posterior wall of left main bronchus

Fig. 4.9e *Endoscopic view of the left main bronchus viewed from halfway down the left main bronchus with the left lower lobe visible distally.*

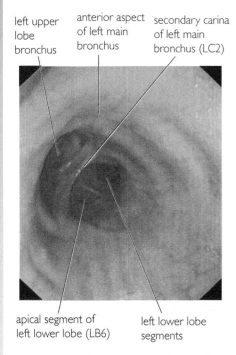

left upper lobe bronchus

anterior aspect of left main bronchus

secondary carina of left main bronchus (LC2)

apical segment of left lower lobe (LB6)

left lower lobe segments

Fig. 4.9f *Endoscopic view of the left main bronchus viewed from two-thirds the way down the left main bronchus, with the left lower lobe visible distally.*

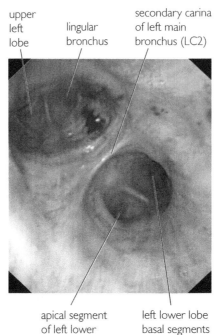

upper left lobe

lingular bronchus

secondary carina of left main bronchus (LC2)

apical segment of left lower lobe (LB6)

left lower lobe basal segments

Fig. 4.9g *Endoscopic view of the left secondary carina with both the upper and lower lobes visible.*

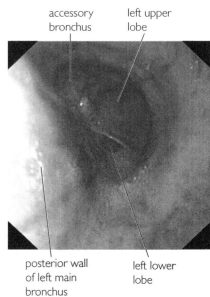

accessory bronchus

left upper lobe

posterior wall of left main bronchus

left lower lobe

Fig. 4.9h *Endoscopic view of the left lower and upper lobes, with the apical segment of the left upper lobe arising from the left main bronchus.*

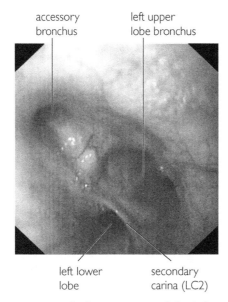

accessory bronchus

left upper lobe bronchus

left lower lobe

secondary carina (LC2)

Fig. 4.9i *Endoscopic view of the left lower and upper lobes with a close view of the apical segment of the left upper lobe arising from the left main bronchus.*

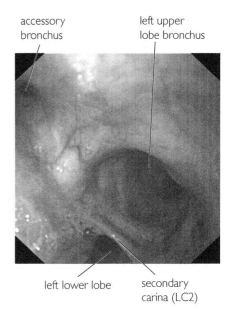

accessory bronchus

left upper lobe bronchus

left lower lobe

secondary carina (LC2)

Fig. 4.9j *Endoscopic view of the left lower and upper lobes with a view of the apical segment of the left upper lobe arising from the left main bronchus, from just above its origin.*

Left upper lobe (Fig. 4.10)

The upper lobe bronchus usually divides into the upper division orifice and the lingual bronchus. The upper division divides into an apicoposterior and anterior bronchus. In the majority of individuals, the apicoposterior bronchus divides into three segmental branches: the apical, posterior and posterolateral branches. In about 15 per cent of individuals the apicoposterior segment has a bipartite structure with the posterolateral subsegment arising from the anterior segment.

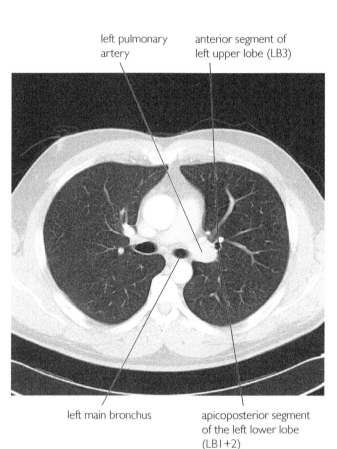

left pulmonary artery

anterior segment of left upper lobe (LB3)

left main bronchus

apicoposterior segment of the left lower lobe (LB1+2)

Fig. 4.10a *Cross-sectional CT scan of the thorax at the level of the left upper lobe bronchus.*

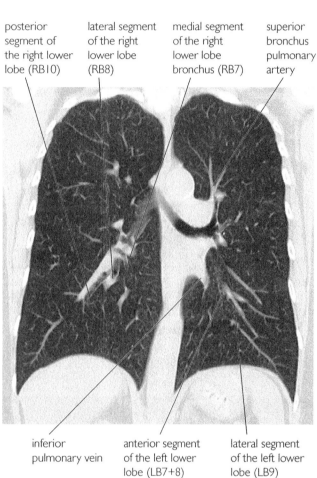

posterior segment of the right lower lobe (RB10)

lateral segment of the right lower lobe (RB8)

medial segment of the right lower lobe bronchus (RB7)

superior bronchus pulmonary artery

inferior pulmonary vein

anterior segment of the left lower lobe (LB7+8)

lateral segment of the left lower lobe (LB9)

Fig. 4.10b *Coronal sectional CT scan of the thorax at the level of the left upper lobe bronchus.*

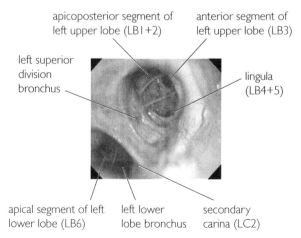

apicoposterior segment of left upper lobe (LB1+2)

anterior segment of left upper lobe (LB3)

left superior division bronchus

lingula (LB4+5)

apical segment of left lower lobe (LB6)

left lower lobe bronchus

secondary carina (LC2)

Fig. 4.10c *Endoscopic view of the left superior bronchus from above the left main bronchial carina.*

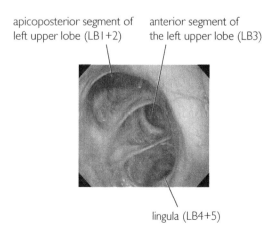

apicoposterior segment of left upper lobe (LB1+2)

anterior segment of the left upper lobe (LB3)

lingula (LB4+5)

Fig. 4.10d *Close-up of the left superior bronchus showing the lingula and left upper lobe segments.*

apicoposterior segment
of the left upper lobe
(LB1+2)

LB3a

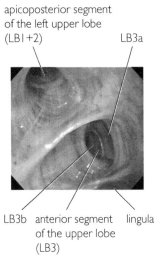

LB3b   anterior segment   lingula
        of the upper lobe
        (LB3)

Fig. 4.10e *Left upper lobe segments showing anterior and apicoposterior segments.*

anterior segment
of the left upper
lobe (LB1)

posterior segment
of the left upper
lobe (LB2)

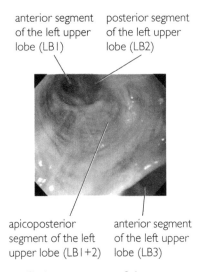

apicoposterior
segment of the left
upper lobe (LB1+2)

anterior segment
of the left upper
lobe (LB3)

Fig. 4.10f *Endoscopic view of the apicoposterior segment of the left upper lobe.*

Lingula (Fig. 4.11)

The lingular bronchus arises from the left upper division bronchus. It divides into superior segmental and inferior segmental branches, which in turn divide into two subsegmental branches. In 25 per cent of individuals, the lingula bifurcates in a lateral and medial fashion. On rare occasions the orifice of the lingula is merged with a segment from the upper lobe.

lingular bronchus   superior segment of   inferior segment
                     the lingula (LB4)   of the lingula (LB5)

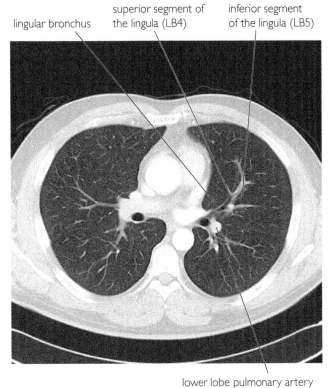

lower lobe pulmonary artery

Fig. 4.11a *Cross-sectional CT scan of the thorax at the level of the lingular bronchus.*

superior pulmonary vein   left upper lobe

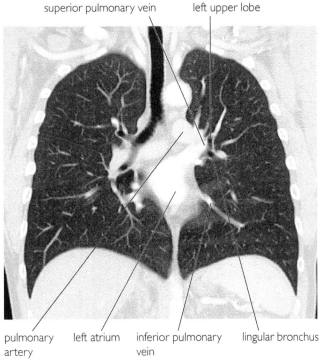

pulmonary   left atrium   inferior pulmonary   lingular bronchus
artery   vein

Fig. 4.11b *Coronal sectional CT scan of the thorax at the level of the lingular bronchus.*

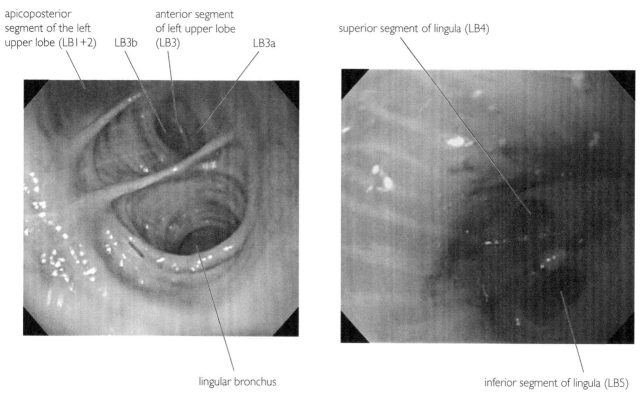

apicoposterior segment of the left upper lobe (LB1+2) LB3b anterior segment of left upper lobe (LB3) LB3a

superior segment of lingula (LB4)

lingular bronchus

inferior segment of lingula (LB5)

Fig. 4.11c *Bronchoscopic view of the lingula and anterior segment of the left upper lobe.*

Fig. 4.11d *Endoscopic view of the lingular segments.*

Left lower lobe (Fig. 4.12)

The left lower lobe bronchus descends posterolaterally and divides into four segments to form the left lower lobe. The apical segment arises about 1 cm after the origin of the left lower lobe bronchus. After a further 1–2 cm the inferior bronchus divides into an anterior basal segmental bronchus and a posterolateral basal bronchus which further bifurcates into lateral basal and posterior basal segments. Endoscopically a prominent secondary carina appears to divide into the apical basal bronchus and the other inferior branches. The most common pattern of division of the left lower lobe is into three branches (tripartite) with separate anterior basal, lateral basal and posterior basal divisions.

superior segment of the lingula (LB4)

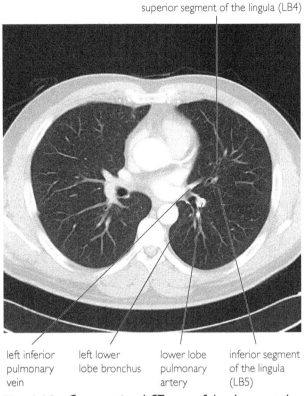

left pulmonary artery

left lower lobe pulmonary artery

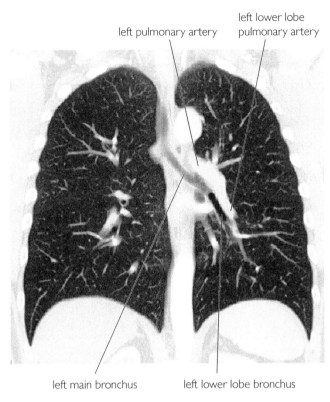

left inferior pulmonary vein

left lower lobe bronchus

lower lobe pulmonary artery

inferior segment of the lingula (LB5)

Fig. 4.12a *Cross-sectional CT scan of the thorax at the level of the left lower lobe bronchus.*

left main bronchus

left lower lobe bronchus

Fig. 4.12b *Coronal sectional CT scan of the thorax at the level of the left lower lobe bronchus.*

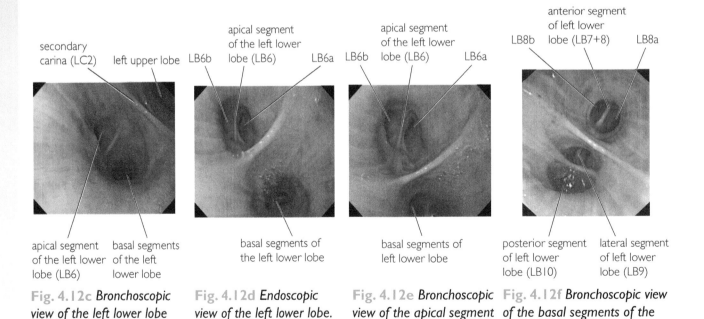

secondary carina (LC2)

left upper lobe

LB6b

apical segment of the left lower lobe (LB6)

LB6a

LB6b

apical segment of the left lower lobe (LB6)

LB6a

anterior segment of left lower lobe (LB7+8)

LB8b

LB8a

apical segment of the left lower lobe (LB6)

basal segments of the left lower lobe

basal segments of the left lower lobe

basal segments of left lower lobe

posterior segment of left lower lobe (LB10)

lateral segment of left lower lobe (LB9)

Fig. 4.12c *Bronchoscopic view of the left lower lobe viewed from just above the left secondary carina.*

Fig. 4.12d *Endoscopic view of the left lower lobe.*

Fig. 4.12e *Bronchoscopic view of the apical segment of the left lower lobe.*

Fig. 4.12f *Bronchoscopic view of the basal segments of the left lower lobe.*

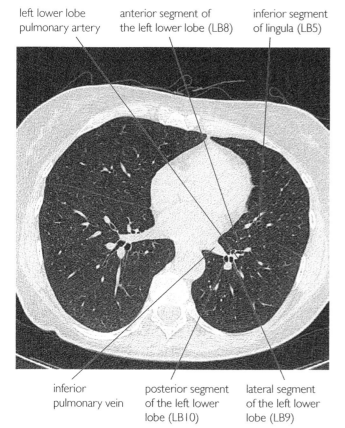

left lower lobe pulmonary artery

anterior segment of the left lower lobe (LB8)

inferior segment of lingula (LB5)

inferior pulmonary vein

posterior segment of the left lower lobe (LB10)

lateral segment of the left lower lobe (LB9)

Fig. 4.12g *Cross-sectional CT scan of the thorax showing the left lower lobe segments.*

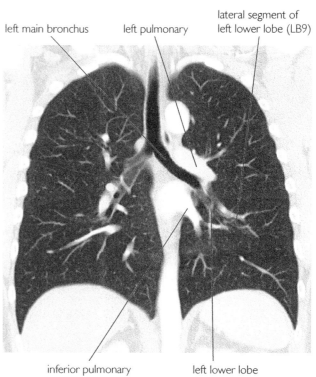

left main bronchus

left pulmonary

lateral segment of left lower lobe (LB9)

inferior pulmonary

left lower lobe

Fig. 4.12h *Coronal sectional CT scan of the thorax showing the left lower lobe segments.*

Vascular relationships and lymph node stations

A good knowledge of the mediastinal anatomy, particularly the relationship between the trachea, bronchial tree and the major vessels, is essential for procedures such as transbronchial needle aspiration (TBNA) and endobronchial ultrasound-guided transbronchial needle aspiration (EBUS-TBNA). The thoracic lymph nodes also have an important role in the staging, and hence treatment, of lung cancer. The anatomy is described in relation to the new International Association for the Study of Lung Cancer (IASLC) lymph node map.

Vascular relationships

The aorta is closely related to the anterior and left lateral aspect of the trachea. The aortic root ascends below the carina and then arches over on the distal aspect of the trachea on the left side and curves around the left hilum (Fig. 5.1).

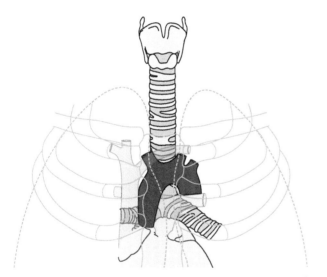

Fig. 5.1a *Relationship to the tracheobronchial tree of the aorta.*

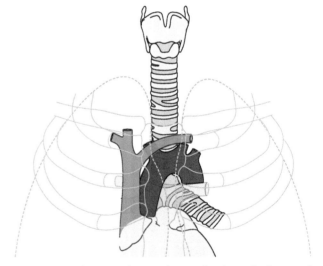

Fig. 5.1b *Relationship to the tracheobronchial tree of the brachiocephalic veins, the superior vena cava and the aorta.*

The left brachiocephalic vein crosses the anterior aspect of the trachea, and its inferior border on the right side of the trachea is at the same level as the aortic arch. It joins with the right brachiocephalic vein and forms the superior vena cava. The superior vena cava crosses the anterior aspect of the right main bronchus and drains into the right atrium.

The pulmonary trunk divides at the level of the carina into the right and left pulmonary arteries (Fig. 5.2). The pulmonary artery trunk is lateral to the aorta, and the right pulmonary artery crosses the infracarinal region and is anterior to the trachea. It is located posterior to the aorta. On the left, the pulmonary artery crosses the anterior aspect of the left main bronchus and then advances behind the left upper lobe, where it divides into superior and inferior branches. The superior branch of the left pulmonary artery is located lateral and posterior to the left upper lobe bronchus. The inferior branch follows the left lower lobe and is lateral and posterior to the left lower lobe. The right pulmonary artery crosses anterior to the right main bronchus and divides into superior and inferior branches lateral to the right main bronchus. The superior branch of the right pulmonary artery is located anterolateral to the right upper lobe bronchus. The inferior branch is sent posterior to the bronchus intermedius and is located posterior and lateral to the right middle lobe and lower lobe branches.

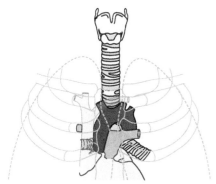

Fig. 5.2a *Relationship to the tracheobronchial tree of the pulmonary arteries.*

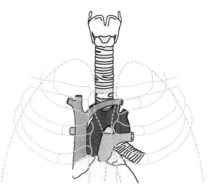

Fig. 5.2b *Relationship to the tracheobronchial tree of the aorta and the pulmonary arteries.*

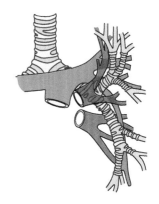

Fig. 5.2c *Relationship to the tracheobronchial tree of the left pulmonary artery.*

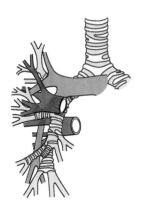

Fig. 5.2d *Relationship to the tracheobronchial tree of the right pulmonary artery.*

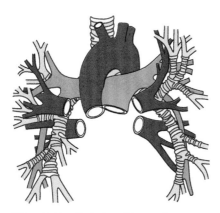

Fig. 5.2e *Relationship to the tracheobronchial tree of the aorta, pulmonary arteries and pulmonary veins.*

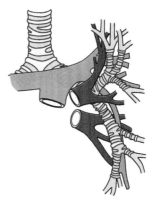

Fig. 5.2f *Relationship to the tracheobronchial tree of the left pulmonary artery (blue) and pulmonary vein (red).*

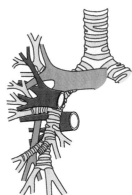

Fig. 5.2g *Relationship to the tracheobronchial tree of the right pulmonary artery (blue) and pulmonary vein (red).*

The pulmonary veins are located anterior and inferior to the pulmonary artery. The superior pulmonary vein is inferior and anterior to the pulmonary artery. On the left side, the superior pulmonary vein is anterior to the left main bronchus, and the branches are predominantly anterior to the bronchi. The inferior pulmonary vein arises in branches that are predominantly posterior to the bronchus and pulmonary arteries, and forms the inferior pulmonary vein medial to the left lower lobe. On the right side, the superior pulmonary vein crosses over anterior to the right main bronchus and the branches arise from the upper and middle lobes. The inferior pulmonary vein on the right side crosses the bronchus intermedius and then travels posterior to the bronchus and pulmonary artery branches.

● Bronchoscopic views

The cross-sectional drawings in Figure 5.3 are from the level of the third to the sixth thoracic vertebral bodies. The drawings give the view that is obtained when looking from above and hence the relationships are those found when performing a bronchoscopy with the patient supine and approached from behind (posterior approach).

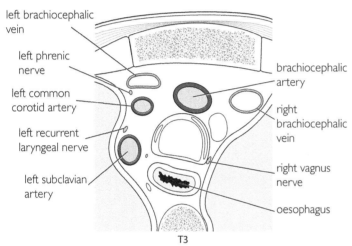

left brachiocephalic vein

left phrenic nerve

left common corotid artery

left recurrent laryngeal nerve

left subclavian artery

brachiocephalic artery

right brachiocephalic vein

right vagnus nerve

oesophagus

T3

Fig. 5.3a *Cross-sectional view at the level of the third vertebral body as viewed from above, showing the main vascular relationships to the trachea.*

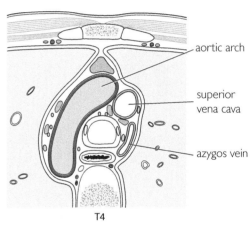

aortic arch

superior vena cava

azygos vein

T4

Fig. 5.3b *Cross-sectional view at the upper level of the fourth vertebral body as viewed from above, showing the main vascular relationships to the trachea.*

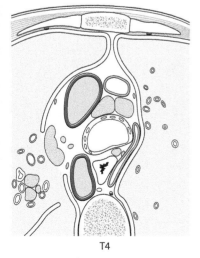

T4

Fig. 5.3c *Cross-sectional view at the lower level of the fourth vertebral body as viewed from above, showing the main vascular relationships to the trachea.*

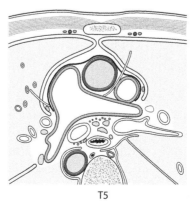

T5

Fig. 5.3d *Cross-sectional view at the level of the fifth vertebral body as viewed from above, showing the main vascular relationships to the main bronchi.*

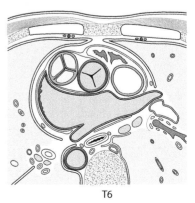

T6

Fig. 5.3e *Cross-sectional view at the level of the sixth vertebral body as viewed from above, showing the main vascular relationships to the main bronchi.*

Lymph node stations

The mediastinal and hilar lymph nodes are described in this section according to the new IASLC classification.

● *Superclavicular zone*

Station 1 (Fig. 5.4)

These are the low cervical, supraclavicular and sternal notch lymph nodes. The upper border is defined as the lower margin of the cricoid cartilage. The lower border is defined by the clavicles and the upper border of the manubrium. Laterality (right or left side) is determined by the midline of the trachea.

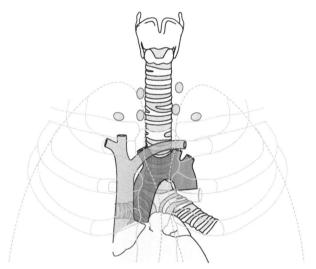

Fig. 5.4a *Station 1 lymph nodes.*

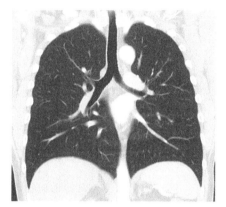

Fig. 5.4b *Coronal section of CT scan depicting margins of the station 1 lymph node zone.*

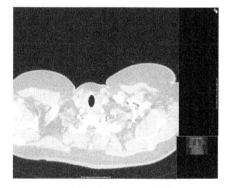

Fig. 5.4c *Axial sections of CT scan depicting the margins of the station 1 lymph node zone: upper margins.*

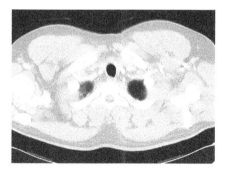

Fig. 5.4d *Axial sections of CT scan depicting the margins of the station 1 lymph node zone: lower margin.*

● Superior mediastinal zone

Station 2: Upper paratracheal lymph nodes (Fig. 5.5)

The upper paratracheal lymph nodes are part of the superior mediastinal zone. The upper border is defined by the apex of the lung to the superior border of the clavicles and manubrium bilaterally. On the right side, the lower border is defined by where the inferior aspect of the brachiocephalic vein crosses the trachea. On the left side, the lower border is defined by the superior border of the aortic arch. The lateral margin is determined by the left lateral border of the trachea so that nodes that are in the anterior aspect of the trachea through to the left lateral margin of the trachea are defined as station 2R lymph nodes, whereas nodes on the left lateral aspect of the trachea are defined as station 2L.

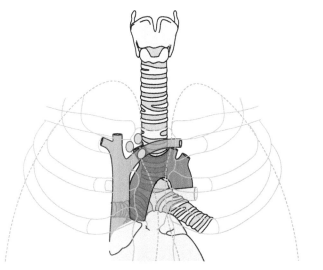

Fig. 5.5a *Station 2R lymph nodes.*

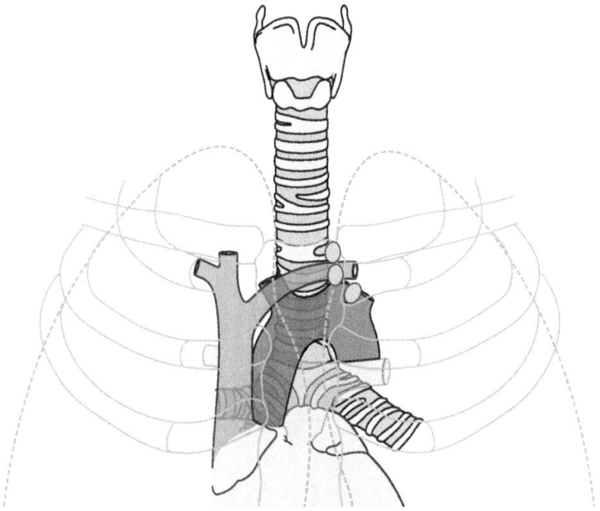

Fig. 5.5b *Station 2L lymph nodes.*

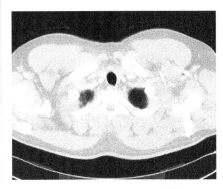

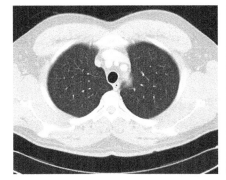

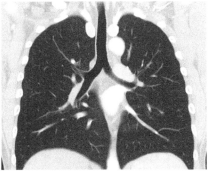

Fig. 5.5c *Axial sections of CT scan depicting the margins of the station 2 lymph node zone: upper margins.*

Fig. 5.5d *Axial sections of CT scan depicting the margins of the station 2 lymph node zone: lower margin.*

Fig. 5.5e *Coronal section of CT scan depicting the margins of the station 2 lymph node zone.*

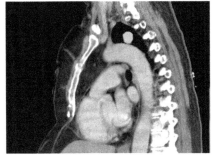

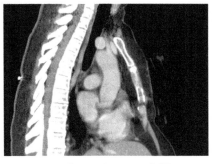

Fig. 5.5f *Sagittal views of CT scan highlighting the station 2 lymph node area: left lateral.*

Fig. 5.5g *Sagittal views of CT scan highlighting the station 2 lymph node area: right lateral.*

Station 3

Station 3A: Prevascular and retrosternal lymph nodes (Fig. 5.6)

The prevascular lymph nodes located on the right side anterior to the superior vena cava up to the sternum. The upper border is defined by the apex of the chest and the lower border at the level of the carina. On the left side, the lymph nodes are anterior to the left carotid artery up to the sternal surface. The upper border is again defined as the apex of the lung and the lower border by the level of the carina. Laterality is defined according to the midline of the trachea.

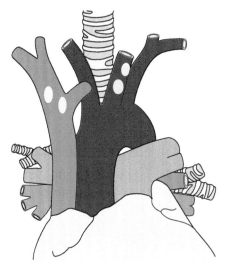

Fig. 5.6a *Station 3a lymph nodes: anterior view.*

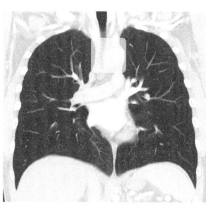

Fig. 5.6b *Station 3a lymph nodes: coronal view.*

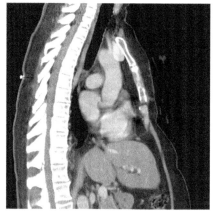

Fig. 5.6c *Sagittal views of CT scan highlighting the station 3a lymph node area: right lateral.*

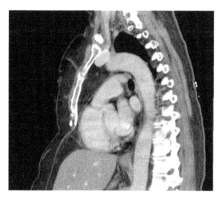

Fig. 5.6d *Sagittal views of CT scan highlighting the station 3a lymph node area: left lateral.*

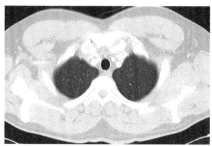

Fig. 5.6e *Axial sections of CT scan depicting the borders of the station 3a lymph node zone: upper border.*

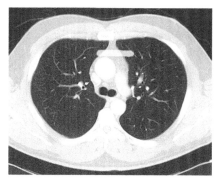

Fig. 5.6f *Axial sections of CT scan depicting the borders of the station 3a lymph node zone: lower border.*

Station 3P: Posterior or retrotracheal lymph nodes (Fig. 5.7)
These are the lymph nodes located posterior to the trachea. The upper margin is defined by the apex of the chest and the lower by the carina.

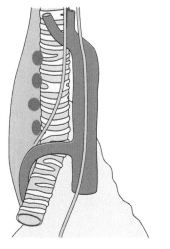

Fig. 5.7a *Station 3p lymph nodes (lateral view).*

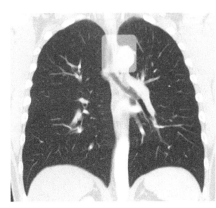

Fig. 5.7b *Coronal view of CT scan depicting the area of the station 3p lymph node.*

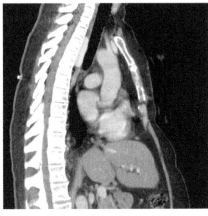

Fig. 5.7c *Sagittal view (right lateral) of CT scan highlighting the station 3p lymph node area.*

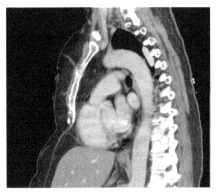

Fig. 5.7d *Sagittal view (left lateral) of CT scan highlighting the station 3p lymph node area.*

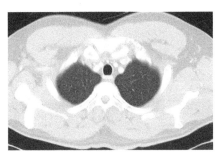

Fig. 5.7e *Axial section of CT scan depicting the upper border of the station 3p lymph node zone.*

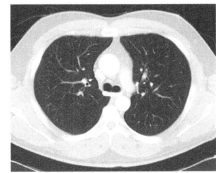

Fig. 5.7f *Axial section of CT scan depicting the lower border of the station 3p lymph node zone.*

Station 4: Lower paratracheal lymph nodes (Fig. 5.8)

The lower right paratracheal lymph nodes include the right paratracheal and anterior carinal lymph nodes. Laterality is defined by the left lateral border of the trachea (2 o'clock position if the midline is considered to be 12 o'clock through to 6 o'clock). The upper border of the 4R lymph nodes is at the level where the lower border of the brachiocephalic vein crosses the trachea. The lower border is defined by the azygos vein. On the left side, the left paratracheal or 4L lymph node is on the left lateral aspect of the trachea from the 2 o'clock position. Its upper border is the upper margin of the aortic arch and the lower border is the upper rim of the left main pulmonary artery.

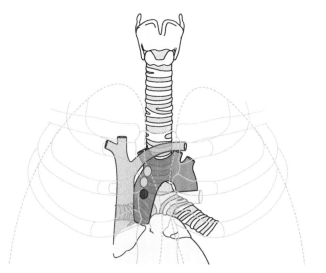

Fig. 5.8a *Station 4R lymph nodes (azygos vein showing lower border).*

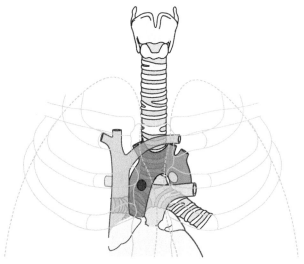

Fig. 5.8b *Station 4L lymph nodes.*

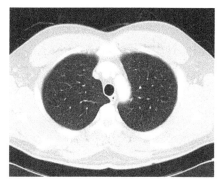

Fig. 5.8c *Axial section of CT scan depicting the upper margins of the station 4 lymph node zone.*

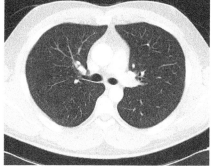

Fig. 5.8d *Axial section of CT scan depicting the lower margin of the station 4 lymph node zone.*

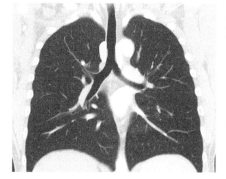

Fig. 5.8e *Coronal section of CT scan depicting the margins of the station 2 lymph node zone.*

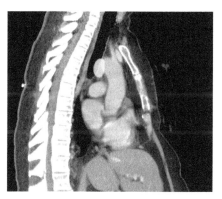

Fig. 5.8f *Sagittal views of CT scan highlighting the margins of the station 4 lymph node zone: right lateral.*

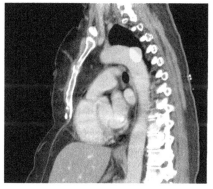

Fig. 5.8g *Sagittal views of CT scan highlighting the margins of the station 4 lymph node zone: left lateral.*

Station 5: Aortic lymph nodes (Fig. 5.9)

These lymph nodes are located on the left side lateral to the ligamentum arteriosum. The upper margin is defined by the lower border of the aortic arch and the lower margin by the upper border of the left main pulmonary artery.

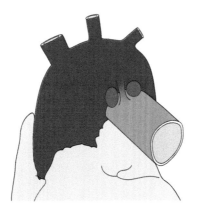

Fig. 5.9a *Station 5 lymph notes: anterior view (nodes in brown).*

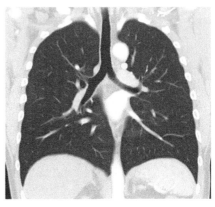

Fig. 5.9b *coronal section of CT scan depicting station 5 lymph nodes.*

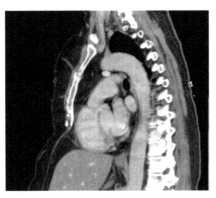

Fig. 5.9c *Sagittal section of CT scan demonstrating station 5 lymph node: left.*

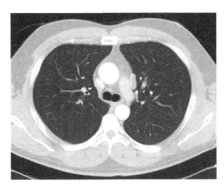

Fig. 5.9d *Axial section of CT scan demonstrating station 5 lymph node.*

Station 6: Para-aortic lymph nodes (Fig. 5.10)

The para-aortic lymph nodes are located on the left side and found anterolateral to the ascending aorta and the aortic arch. The upper border is a horizontal line through the upper border of the aortic arch and the lower border defined by the lower level of the aortic arch.

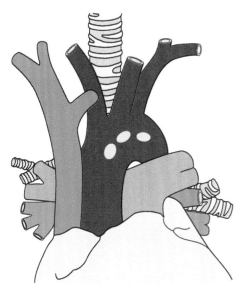

Fig. 5.10a *Station 6 lymph nodes: anterior view.*

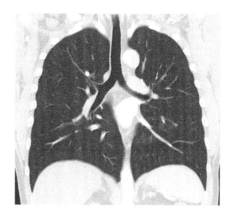

Fig. 5.10b *Station 6 lymph nodes: coronal view.*

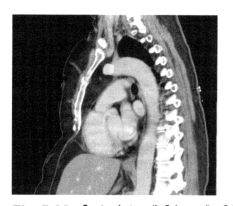

Fig. 5.10c *Sagittal view (left lateral) of CT scan depicting the station 6 lymph node.*

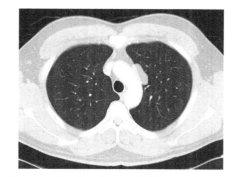

Fig. 5.10d *Axial view of CT scan depicting the station 6 lymph node.*

Inferior mediastinal nodes

Station 7: Subcarinal lymph nodes (Fig. 5.11)

These are the lymph nodes located below the main carina of the trachea. The lower border is defined by the lower border of the bronchus intermedius on the right side and the lower border of the left main bronchus on the left side.

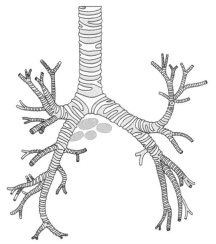

Fig. 5.11a *Station 7 lymph nodes.*

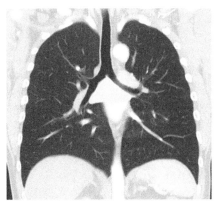

Fig. 5.11b *Coronal section of CT scan depicting the margins of the station 7 lymph node zone.*

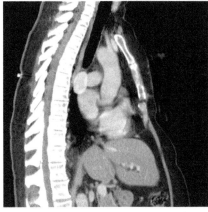

Fig. 5.11c *Sagittal views of CT scan depicting the station 7 lymph node: right lateral.*

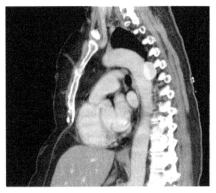

Fig. 5.11d *Sagittal views of CT scan depicting the station 7 lymph node: left lateral.*

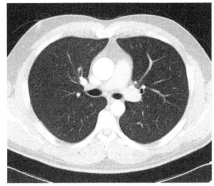

Fig. 5.11e *Axial section of CT scan depicting the upper margins of the station 7 lymph node zone.*

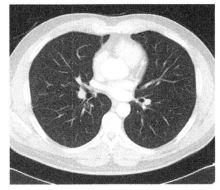

Fig. 5.11f *Axial section of CT scan depicting the lower margins of the station 7 lymph node zone.*

Lower zone

Station 8: Para-oesophageal lymph nodes (Fig. 5.12)

These are lymph nodes lying adjacent to the wall of the oesophagus. They are the nodes located below the sub-carinal lymph nodes. Hence the upper border on the right side is defined by the lower border of the bronchus intermedius and the left by the lower border of the left main bronchus. The inferior extent of the lymph nodes is the dome of the diaphragm.

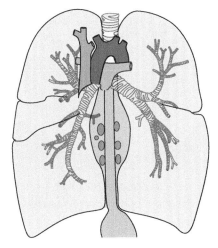

Fig. 5.12a *Station 8 lymph nodes.*

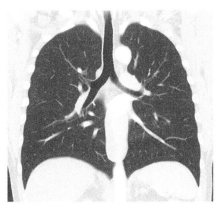

Fig. 5.12b *Coronal section of CT scan depicting the margins of the station 8 lymph node zone.*

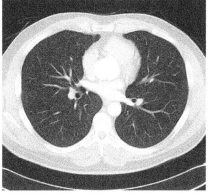

Fig. 5.12c *Axial section of CT scan depicting the upper margins of the station 8 lymph node zone.*

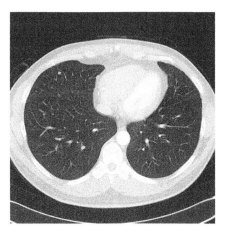

Fig. 5.12d *Axial section of CT scan depicting the lower margins of the station 8 lymph node zone.*

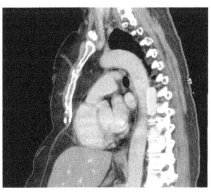

Fig. 5.12e *Sagittal views of CT scan depicting the station 8 lymph node: left lateral.*

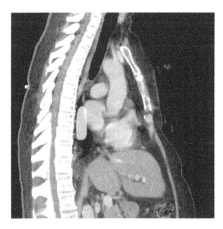

Fig. 5.12f *Sagittal views of CT scan depicting the station 8 lymph node: right lateral.*

Station 9: Pulmonary ligament lymph nodes (Fig. 5.13)

The pulmonary ligament lymph nodes are located along the pulmonary ligament. The upper border of station 9 is defined by the inferior pulmonary vein and the lower border by the diaphragm.

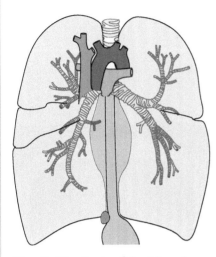

Fig. 5.13a *Station 9 lymph nodes.*

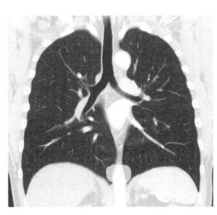

Fig. 5.13b *Coronal section of CT scan depicting the lower margins of the station 9 lymph node zone.*

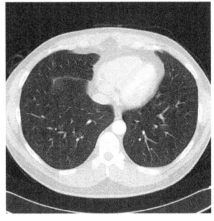

Fig. 5.13c *Axial section of CT scan depicting the upper margins of the station 9 lymph node zone.*

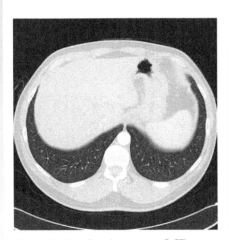

Fig. 5.13d *Axial section of CT scan depicting the lower margins of station 9 lymph node zone.*

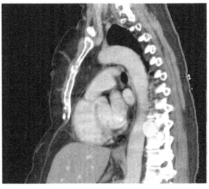

Fig. 5.13e *Sagittal views of CT scan depicting the station 9 lymph node: left lateral.*

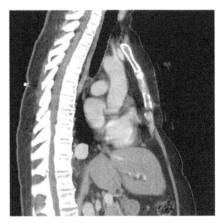

Fig. 5.13f *Sagittal views of CT scan depicting the station 9 lymph node: right lateral.*

● *Hilar/interlobar zone (hilar nodes)*

Station 10: Main bronchial lymph nodes (Fig. 5.14)

Station 10 or hilar lymph nodes are found adjacent to the right and left main bronchi and the main pulmonary artery and pulmonary vein. On the right side, the upper border is determined by the lower rim of the azygos vein down to the distal margin of the right main bronchus. On the left side, the lymph nodes are located between the upper rim of the pulmonary artery and the lower aspect of the left main bronchus.

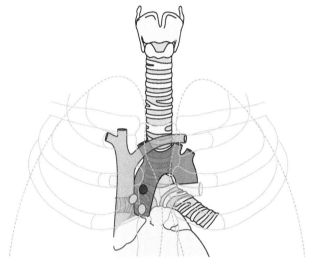

Fig. 5.14a *Station 10R lymph nodes (azygos vein depicting upper margin).*

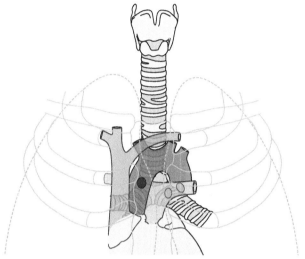

Fig. 5.14b *Station 10L lymph nodes.*

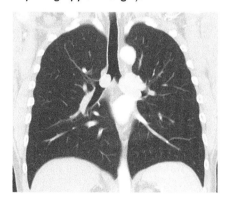

Fig. 5.14c *Coronal view of CT scan depicting the margins of the station 10 lymph node zone.*

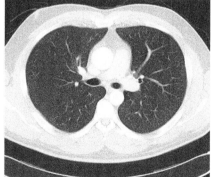

Fig. 5.14d *Axial sections of CT scan depicting the margins of the station 10 lymph node zone: upper margins.*

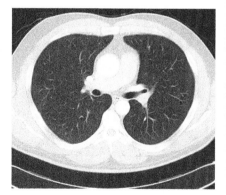

Fig. 5.14e *Axial sections of CT scan depicting the margins of the station 10 lymph node zone: lower margins.*

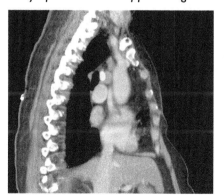

Fig. 5.14f *Sagittal section of CT scan depicting the station 10R (right) lymph node.*

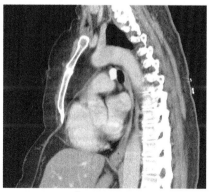

Fig. 5.14g *Sagittal section of CT scan (left lateral) depicting the station 10L (left) lymph node zone.*

Station 11: Interlobar lymph nodes (Fig. 5.15)

These interlobar lymph nodes are located between the origin of the lobar bronchus. On the right side are the superior station 11 lymph nodes (11Rs), which are located between the right upper lobe and the bronchus intermedius. The inferior station 11 lymph nodes (11Ri) are located between the middle lobe bronchus and the lower lobe bronchus. On the left side, the station 11 lymph nodes (11L) are located between the left superior division bronchus and the left lower lobe bronchus.

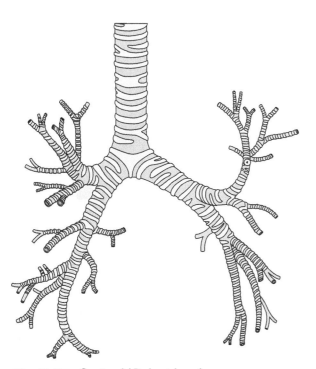

Fig. 5.15a *Station 11Rs lymph nodes.*

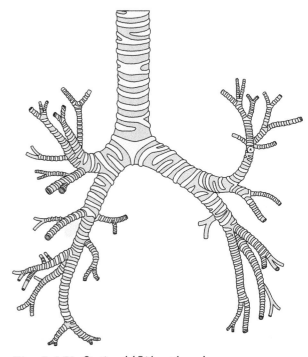

Fig. 5.15b *Station 11Ri lymph nodes.*

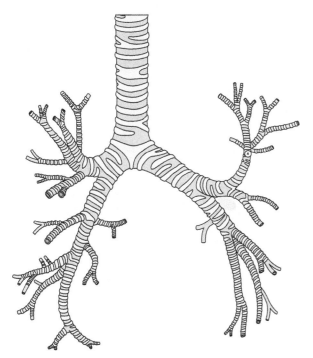

Fig. 5.15c *Station 11L lymph nodes.*

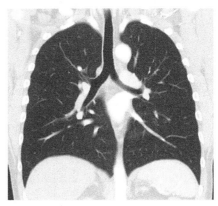

Fig. 5.15d *Coronal view of CT scan depicting the station 11 lymph nodes.*

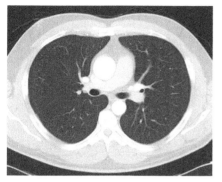

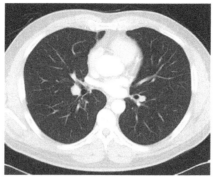

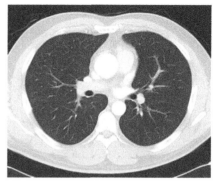

Fig. 5.15e *Axial section of CT scan depicting Station 11Rs lymph node.*

Fig. 5.15f *Axial sections of CT scan depicting: station 11Ri lymph node.*

Fig. 5.15g *Axial sections of CT scan depicting: station 11L lymph node.*

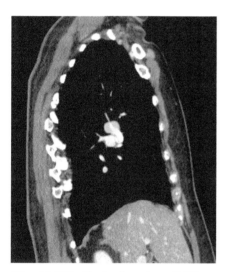

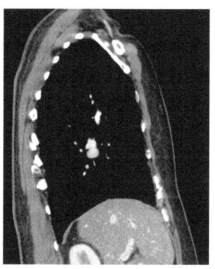

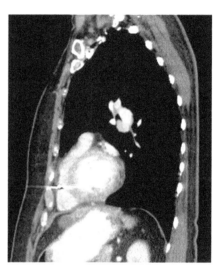

Fig. 5.15h *Sagittal section of CT scan (right lateral) depicting the station 11Rs (right) lymph node.*

Fig. 5.15i *Sagittal section of CT scan (right lateral) depicting the station 11R (right) lymph node.*

Fig. 5.15j *Sagittal section of CT scan (left lateral) depicting the station 11L (left) lymph node.*

● *Peripheral zone*

Stations 12, 13 and 14

These are the lymph nodes located adjacent to the lobar bronchi (station 12) nodes, adjacent to the upper lobes (12u), middle lobe (12m) and lower lobes (12l). The station 13 lymph nodes are segmental nodes and the station 14 nodes are located adjacent to the subsegmental bronchi. These lymph nodes are not accessible at bronchoscopy and are therefore not discussed further.

Transbronchial fine-needle aspiration (anterior approach)

Transbronchial fine-needle aspiration (TBNA) is a simple, cheap technique for sampling mediastinal nodes. Hilar lymph nodes, masses adjacent to the airways and submucosal disease may also be sampled with this technique. A variety of needles are available but the needle should be retractable with a length of between 13 and 15 mm and a gauge of between 18 and 22 (Fig. 6.1).

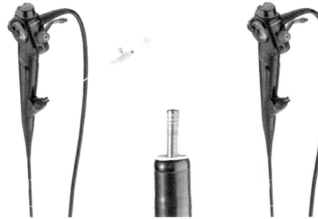
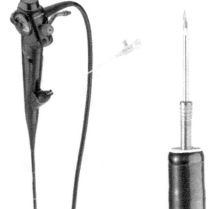

Fig. 6.1a *Bronchoscope with transbronchial fine-needle aspiration needle: withdrawn into the sheath.*

Fig. 6.1b *Bronchoscope with transbronchial fine-needle aspiration needle: extended out of the sheath.*

Planning/site selection

The computed tomography (CT) scan of the thorax should be examined prior to TBNA and the site of aspiration should be predetermined (Fig. 6.2a). The simplest approach is to relate the airway to a clock face and plan the position of target sites in this manner (Fig. 6.2b). The CT scan is obtained by imaging from the feet upwards (Fig. 6.2c), whereas at bronchoscopy the patient is approached from the head downwards (Fig. 6.2d). It is therefore important to account for these differences. For patients who are being approached from the anterior side, the simple trick is to flip the image in the horizontal axis (Fig. 6.2e). The vertical position also needs to be determined and can be described in terms of cartilage spaces or rings above and below the carina (Fig. 6.2f). In some cases it may be necessary to relate the vertical position to the origin of the segmental bronchi. More detailed descriptions are given for the example lymph node stations in this chapter, but it should be emphasized that this is merely a guide and individual sites for aspiration are determined according to the patient's CT scan. Modern multi-planar reformatting of CTs and software modules with virtual bronchoscopy (Fig. 6.2g) and lymph node highlighting (Fig. 6.2h) may help to determine the site of needle aspiration.

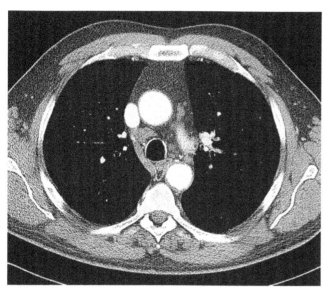

Fig. 6.2a *CT scan with right paratracheal lymph node present.*

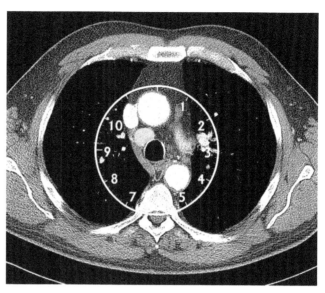

Fig. 6.2b *CT scan with the right paratracheal lymph node highlighted in yellow and the clock face showing that the lymph node is in 10–11 o'clock position.*

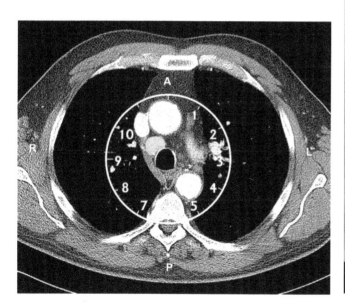

Fig. 6.2c *Cross-sectional CT scan of the thorax; note the relative position of the anterior and posterior aspects of the patient.*

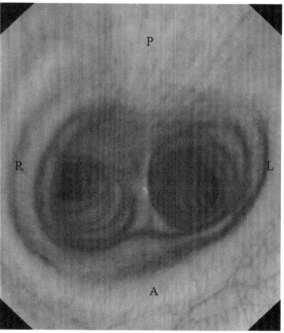

Fig. 6.2d *Bronchoscopic view; note the relative position of the anterior and posterior aspects of the patient.*

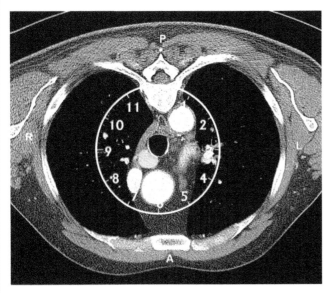

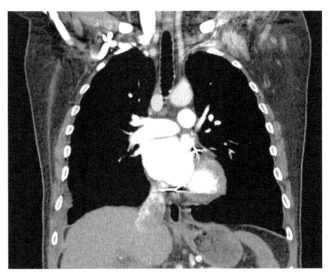

Fig. 6.2e *Cross-sectional CT scan of the thorax flipped on the horizontal axis so as to align the anterior and posterior aspects of the patient with the bronchoscopic view.*

Fig. 6.2f *Coronal CT reformat to help determine the vertical position of the lymph node in relation to the carina.*

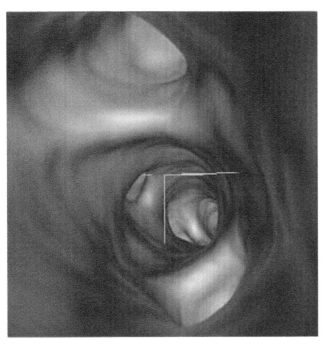

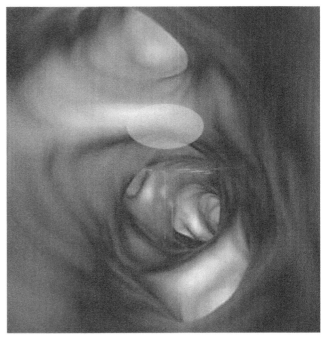

Fig. 6.2g *Virtual bronchoscopy derived from CT scanning.*

Fig. 6.2h *Virtual bronchoscopy derived from CT scanning with lymph node highlighting.*

Technique

Transbronchial fine-needle aspiration should be performed first during the bronchoscopy and, in the case of mediastinal lymph node sampling, before inspection of the airways. Minimal use of suction should be employed in order to minimize the risk of aspirating cellular material from the distal airways, which may lead to false-positive results. These simple precautions virtually prevent any false-positive results. This is important in the staging of lung cancer where a false-positive result would upstage a patient and deny him or her potentially curative surgery. It is also important to sample the highest-stage lymph nodes first, e.g. N3 lymph nodes followed by N2 lymph nodes and finally N1 lymph nodes. The needle should be inserted through the instrument channel of the bronchoscope with the bronchoscope as straight as possible in the trachea. Any flexion or extension of the distal portion of the scope should be avoided until the hub of the needle is outside the bronchoscope. This is essential in order to minimize bronchoscope damage.

A number of techniques can be used to sample the lymph node (Fig. 6.3):

- jabbing
- piggyback
- cough.

● Jabbing technique

This involves guiding the bronchoscope to the target area and then apposing the distal hub of the needle to the airway wall. The distal portion of the scope should be angulated to ensure that the needle penetrates through the airway as perpendicular as possible. There should be an angle of at least 45° between the airway wall and the needle. The

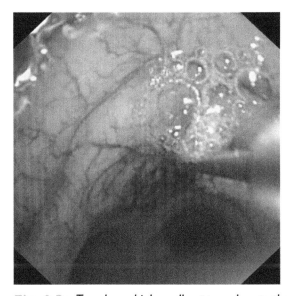

Fig. 6.3a *Transbronchial needle apposed on to the airway wall at an angle of at least 45° in the anterior carinal position.*

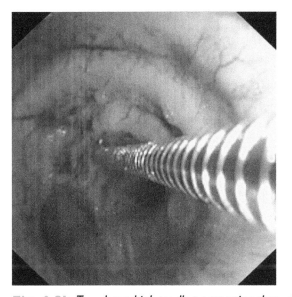

Fig. 6.3b *Transbronchial needle penetrating through the airway wall in the anterior carinal position.*

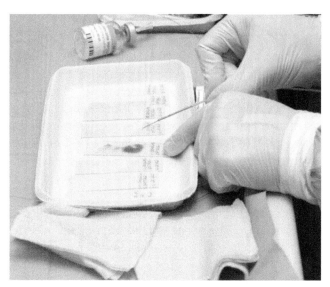

Fig. 6.3c *Cytology slides being prepared from aspirates. The aspirate is first sprayed on to the slides and then thin smears are made.*

needle is then pushed through the airway wall and gently manipulated back and forth. At the same time, an assistant should apply suction at the proximal end of the TBNA needle with a 20 mL syringe. The samples collected are then smeared on to slides and sprayed with a fixative, or alternatively injected into saline or cytolyte solution, depending on the preference of the local site pathologist. Any tissue fragments or slivers obtained are placed in formalin and sent for histological analysis. The availability of rapid on-site cytological evaluation (ROSE) significantly reduces the time of the procedure and improves diagnostic yield.

In the absence of a ROSE, at least four needle passes are made at each target site when assessing patients with suspected lung cancer. The site with the highest possible lymph node stage should be sampled first, then moving progressively down to the lower site.

● *Piggyback method*

With this method the needle is advanced, and once the hub is protruding through the distal end, the needle is fixed by pressing the insertion port of the bronchoscope with an index finger. This does cause the catheter to bend at this point and the technique is better reserved for single-use disposable needles. Once the needle is fixed into position, the scope and the needle can be moved in unison and pushed forward at the desired location until the needle penetrates the airway wall. The needle is moved back and forth with an assistant applying suction as described for the jabbing technique.

● *Cough technique*

This method employs either of the above approaches in conjunction with a controlled cough to facilitate penetration of the needle through the airway wall. It relies on patient cooperation and may not always be successful.

Lymph node stations

It is possible to sample any of the lymph nodes that are adjacent to the airways using TBNA. The lymph node stations are described according to the new International Association for the Study of Lung Cancer (IASLC) classification.

● *Superior mediastinal lymph nodes: upper zone*

Station 4R: Lower right paratracheal lymph node (Fig. 6.4)

The station 4R or right paratracheal lymph node is classically located in the right anterior aspect of the trachea. The exact position should be predetermined from the CT scan. Usually on the CT scan the right paratracheal lymph node is located in the 10–11 o'clock position, if the anterior midline is considered to be 12 o'clock. However, one should note that the CT scans are obtained by looking at the patient from the feet upwards; but when patients undergo a bronchoscopy, the airways are viewed with the head downwards. When the patient is approached from the front, with the patient in a semi-recumbent position, the posterior wall is now at the 12 o'clock position and the anterior wall at the 6 o'clock position. Hence, in this position the right paratracheal lymph node is now positioned between the seven and 8 o'clock positions. The simplest way is to flip the CT scan in the horizontal axis. The bronchoscopic position of the right paratracheal lymph node is between seven and 8 o'clock. Bending the bronchoscope posteriorly in this position is more difficult. Easier and more accurate access can be achieved by rotating the bronchoscope by about 180°. The lymph node is now in the one to 2 o'clock position. The vertical position of the right paratracheal lymph node is about two to four intercartilage spaces above the carina.

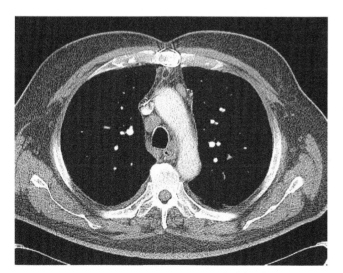

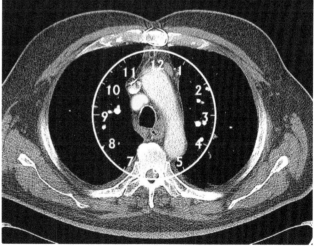

Fig. 6.4a *Cross-sectional CT scan of the thorax at the level of the aortic arch showing a station 4R lymph node.*

Fig. 6.4b *Cross-sectional CT scan with a superimposed clock face and a station 4R lymph node highlighted in yellow.*

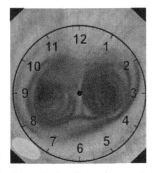

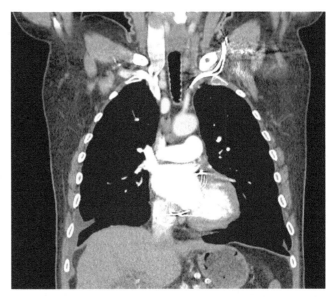

Fig. 6.4c *Cross-sectional CT scan of the thorax flipped on the horizontal axis. The 4R lymph node is in the 7–8 o'clock position.*

Fig. 6.4d *Coronal section of CT scan showing the vertical position of the lymph node, which is usually about two to four rings above the carina.*

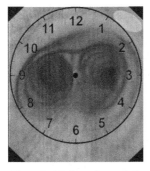

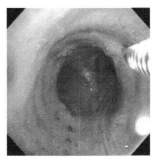

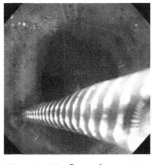

Fig. 6.4e *Bronchoscopic view of the station 4R lymph node which is in the 7–8 o'clock position about two to four intercartilage spaces above the carina.*

Fig. 6.4f *Rotation of the bronchoscope by 180° facilitates access of the station 4R lymph node which is now in the 1–2 o'clock position.*

Fig. 6.4g *Bronchoscopic view of the needle inserted into a 4R lymph node in the 2 o'clock position with the scope rotated anteriorly by 180°.*

Fig. 6.4h *Bronchoscopic view of the needle inserted into a 4R lymph node in the 8 o'clock position with the scope in the neutral position.*

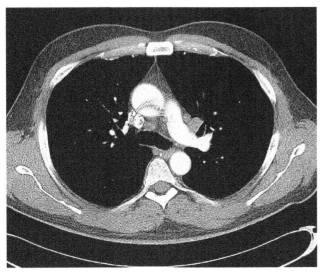

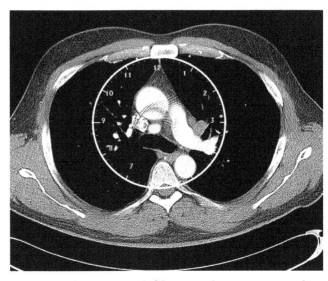

Fig. 6.4i *Cross-sectional CT scan of anterior carinal lymph node (station 4R) anterior to the carina.*

Fig. 6.4j *Cross-sectional CT scan with a superimposed clock face and anterior carinal lymph node (station 4R) highlighted in yellow.*

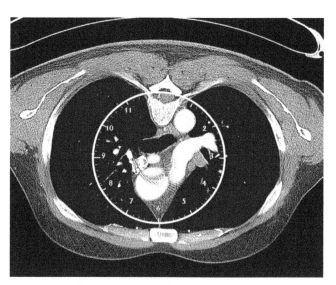

Fig. 6.4k *Cross-sectional CT scan flipped on the horizontal axis. The anterior carinal lymph node (station 4R) is in the 6–6.30 o'clock position.*

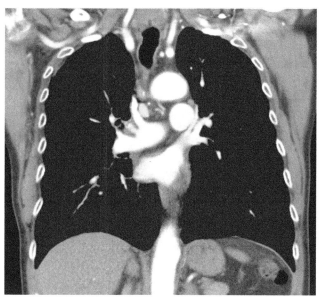

Fig. 6.4l *Coronal section of CT scan showing the vertical position of the anterior carinal lymph node which is usually at the level of the carina.*

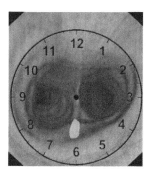

Fig. 6.4m *Bronchoscopic view of the station 4R (anterior carinal) lymph node which is in the 6 o'clock position at the level of the carina.*

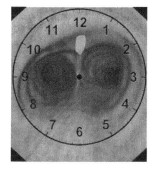

Fig. 6.4n *Rotation of the bronchoscope by 180° facilitates access of the station 4R (anterior carinal) lymph node, which is now in the 12 o'clock position.*

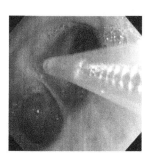

Fig. 6.4o *Bronchoscopic view of needle inserted into a 4R lymph node in the 12 o'clock position with the scope rotated anteriorly by 180°.*

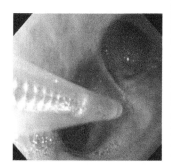

Fig. 6.4p *Bronchoscopic view of the needle inserted into a 4R lymph node in the 6 o'clock position with the scope in the neutral position.*

As described in Chapter 5, station 4R can extend anterior to the trachea through to the 2 o'clock position. Nodes located anterior to the trachea were previously described as anterior carinal lymph nodes. They are usually located in the 11.30 to 12 o'clock position on the CT scan. At bronchoscopy this relates to the 6–6.30 position when the patient is being approached from the front. During TBNA when the patient is being approached from the front, it is easier to sample the lymph nodes if the scope is rotated by 180° so that the lymph node is now in an anterior direction of the bronchoscope.

Station 4L: Lower left paratracheal lymph node (Fig. 6.5)

The station 4L or left paratracheal lymph node is located on the left lateral position of the trachea at or above the level of the carina. On the CT scan the lymph node is located in the 3 o'clock position. When the patient is being approached from the front at bronchoscopy, the lymph node is located at the same 3 o'clock position. The vertical position of the lymph node is at the level of the carina or one space above. In practice this lymph node is more easily accessed by rotating the bronchoscope 90° in an anticlockwise direction. Once the needle has penetrated the airway wall, the torsion on the bronchoscope can be relaxed and the needle moved back while the bronchoscope is in the neutral position (as in Fig. 6.5h).

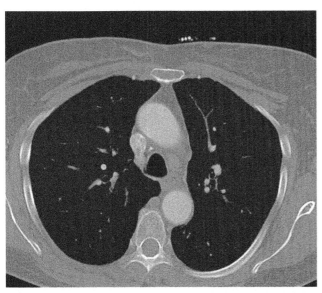

Fig. 6.5a *Cross-sectional CT scan of the thorax showing a station 4L lymph node.*

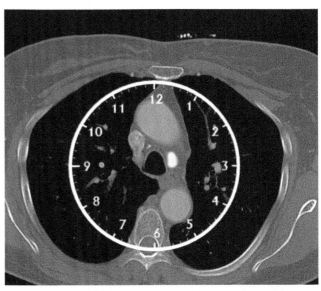

Fig. 6.5b *Cross-sectional CT scan with a superimposed clockface and a station 4L lymph node highlighted in yellow.*

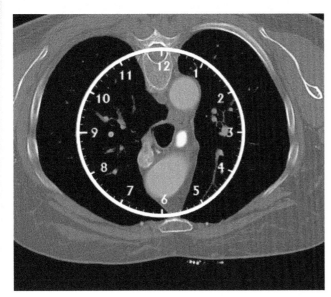

Fig. 6.5c *Cross-sectional CT scan of the thorax flipped on the horizontal axis. The 4L lymph node is in the 3 o'clock position.*

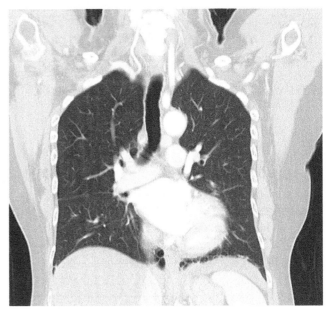

Fig. 6.5d *Coronal section of CT scan showing the vertical position of the station 4L lymph node, which is usually at one intercartilage space above the carina.*

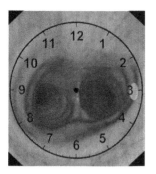

Fig. 6.5e *Bronchoscopic view of the station 4L lymph node which is in the 3 o'clock position about one intercartilage space above the carina.*

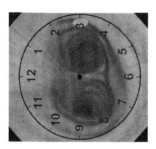

Fig. 6.5f *Rotation of the bronchoscope by 90° anticlockwise facilitates access of the station 4L lymph node.*

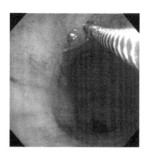

Fig. 6.5g *Bronchoscopic view of the needle inserted into a 4L lymph node with the scope rotated anticlockwise by 90°.*

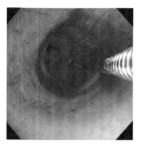

Fig. 6.5h *Bronchoscopic view of the needle inserted into a 4L lymph node in the 3 o'clock position with the scope in the neutral position.*

Station 3P: Posterior tracheal lymph node (Fig. 6.6)

The posterior carinal lymph node is usually located at the level of the carina on the posterior aspect of the trachea. On CT terms it can be considered to be in the 5.30–6 o'clock position. At bronchoscopy it is located at the level of the carina in the 12–12.30 o'clock position when the patient is approached from the front. The forward angulation of the bronchoscope is greater in the anterior direction and therefore access for TBNA is improved by rotating the scope to 180° so that the lymph nodes are now anterior in the 12–12.30 o'clock position. The seventh edition of the IASLC staging classification regards all lymph nodes posterior to the trachea as station 3p, so the site of needle sampling should be planned from the CT scan of the thorax.

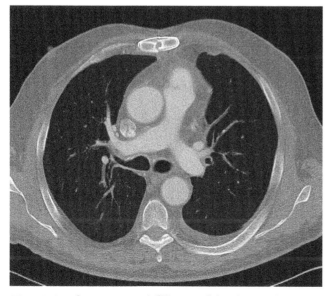

Fig. 6.6a *Cross-sectional CT scan of the thorax showing a station 3p lymph node.*

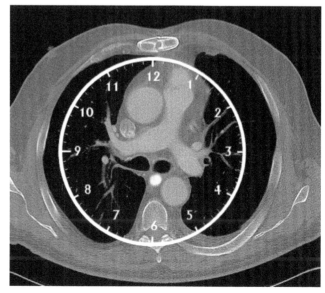

Fig. 6.6b *Cross-sectional CT scan with a superimposed clockface and a station 3p lymph node highlighted in yellow.*

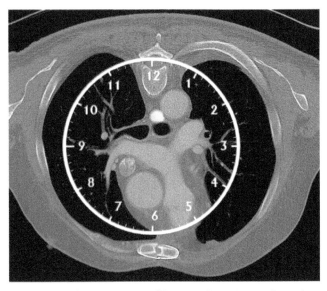

Fig. 6.6c *Cross-sectional CT scan of the thorax flipped on the horizontal axis. The 3p lymph node is in the 12–12.30 o'clock position.*

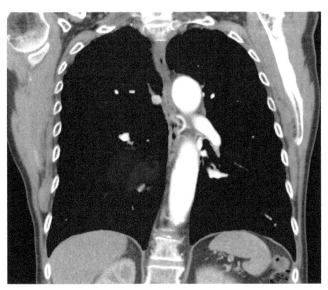

Fig. 6.6d *Coronal section of CT scan showing the vertical position of the station 3p lymph node, which is usually at the level of the carina.*

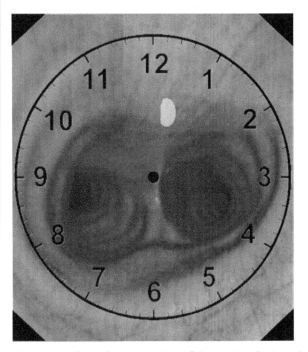

Fig. 6.6e *Bronchoscopic view of the station 3p lymph node which is in the 12–12.30 o'clock position about one intercartilage space above the carina.*

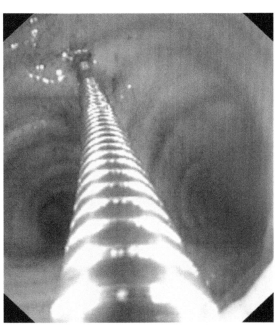

Fig. 6.6f *Bronchoscopic view of needle inserted into a 3p lymph node in the 12 o'clock position with the scope in the neutral position.*

● *Inferior mediastinal lymph nodes*

Station 7: Subcarinal lymph node (Fig. 6.7)

The station 7 or subcarinal lymph nodes are located just inferior to the carina. The carina is composed of three bundles of cartilage and ligament and hence direct puncture through the carina tends to be unsuccessful. The subcarinal lymph nodes should be approached in the right main bronchus by one space below the carina. On the CT scan this translates to the 3 o'clock position and is the same if the patient is being approached from the front. Easier and more accurate access is facilitated by rotating the bronchoscope by 90° anticlockwise.

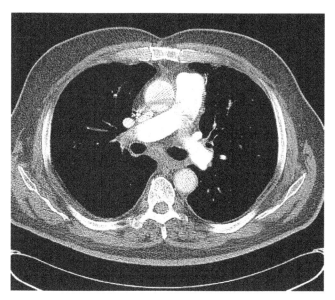

Fig. 6.7a *Cross-sectional CT scan of the thorax showing a station 7 lymph node.*

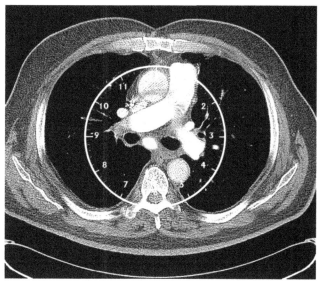

Fig. 6.7b *Cross-sectional CT scan with a superimposed clock face and a station 7 lymph node highlighted in yellow.*

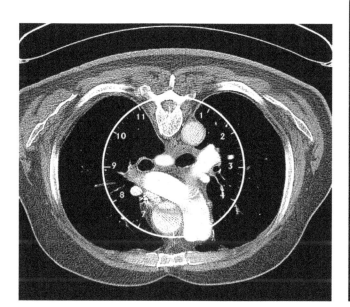

Fig. 6.7c *Cross-sectional CT scan of the thorax flipped on the horizontal axis. The station 7 lymph node is in the 3 o'clock position.*

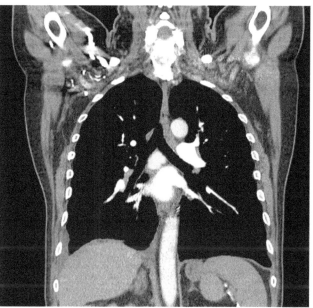

Fig. 6.7d *Coronal section of CT scan showing the vertical position of the station 7 lymph node which is usually one intercartilage space below the carina in the right main bronchus.*

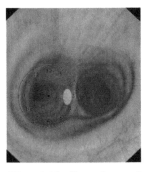

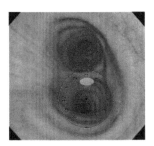

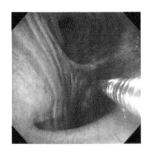

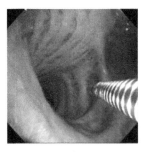

Fig. 6.7e *Bronchoscopic view of the station 4L lymph node which is in the 3 o'clock position one intercartilage space below the carina in the right main bronchus.*

Fig. 6.7f *Rotation of the bronchoscope by 90° anticlockwise facilitates access of the station 7 lymph node.*

Fig. 6.7g *Bronchoscopic view of needle inserted into a station 7 lymph node with the scope rotated anticlockwise by 90°.*

Fig. 6.7h *Bronchoscopic view of the needle inserted into a station 7 lymph node in the 3 o'clock position with the scope in the neutral position.*

● Hilar zone lymph nodes

Station 10R: Right main bronchial lymph node (Fig. 6.8)

The station 10R or right main bronchial lymph node is located anterior to the right main bronchus about one intercartilage space below the carina in the 12 o'clock position on the CT scan. Where the patient is being bronchoscoped from the front, this is equivalent to the 6 o'clock position in the right main bronchus one space below the carina. Again, for improved access when performing TBNA, the bronchoscope should be rotated by 180° so that the lymph node is now positioned anteriorly at the 12 o'clock position.

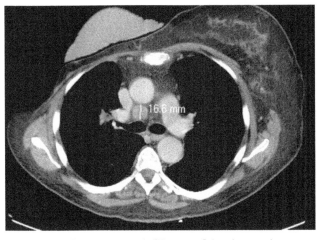

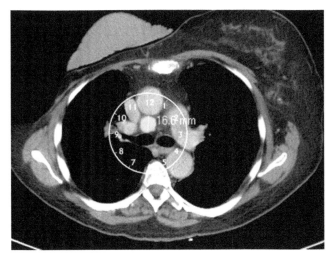

Fig. 6.8a *Cross-sectional CT scan of the thorax showing a station 10R lymph node.*

Fig. 6.8b *Cross-sectional CT scan with a superimposed clock face and a station 10R lymph node highlighted in yellow.*

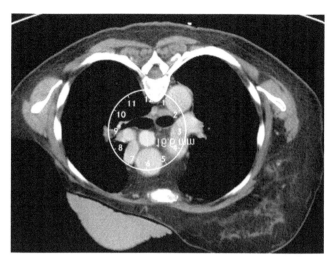

Fig. 6.8c *Cross-sectional CT scan of the thorax flipped on the horizontal axis. The 10R lymph node is in the 6 o'clock position in the right main bronchus.*

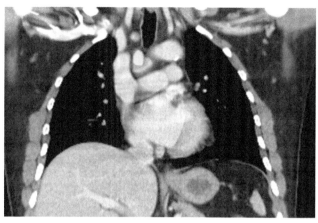

Fig. 6.8d *Coronal section of CT scan showing the vertical position of the station 10R lymph node which is usually one intercartilage space below the carina in the right main bronchus.*

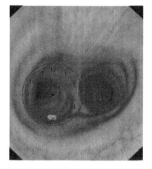 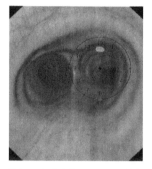 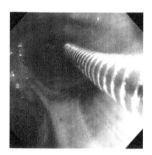 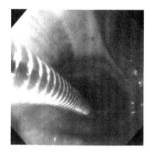

Fig. 6.8e *Bronchoscopic view of the station 10R lymph node which is in the 6 o'clock position about one intercartilage space below the carina in the right main bronchus.*

Fig. 6.8f *Rotation of the bronchoscope by 180° clockwise facilitates access of the station 10R lymph node.*

Fig. 6.8g *Bronchoscopic view of the needle inserted into a 10R lymph node with the scope rotated clockwise by 180°.*

Fig. 6.8h *Bronchoscopic view of the needle inserted into a station 10R lymph node in the 6 o'clock position with the scope in the neutral position.*

Station 10L: Left main bronchial lymph node (Fig. 6.9)

The left main bronchial lymph node is located on the anterior aspect of the left main bronchus approximately one interspace below the carina in the 12 o'clock position. During bronchoscopy when the patient is being approached from the front, the lymph node is in the 6 o'clock position and again access improved by rotating the scope through 180° so that the approach is now in the 12 o'clock position.

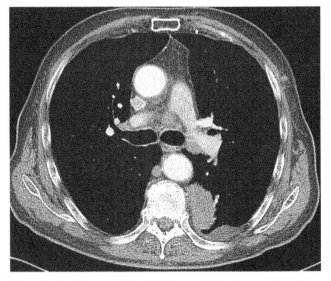

Fig. 6.9a *Cross-sectional CT scan of the thorax showing a station 10L lymph node.*

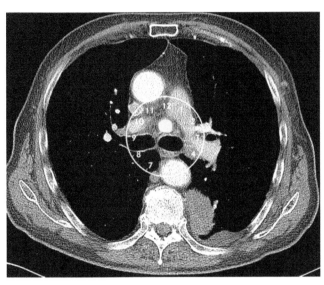

Fig. 6.9b *Cross-sectional CT scan with a superimposed clock face and a station 10L lymph node highlighted in yellow in the 6 o'clock position.*

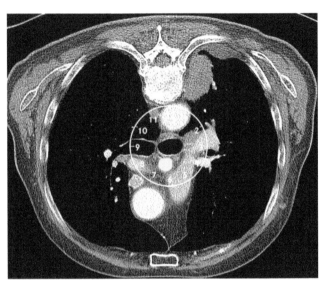

Fig. 6.9c *Cross-sectional CT scan of the thorax flipped on the horizontal axis. The 10L lymph node is in the 12 o'clock position.*

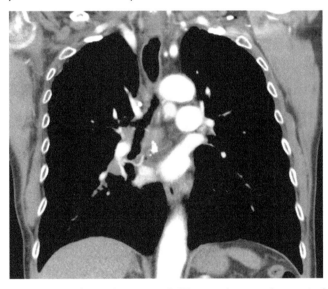

Fig. 6.9d *Coronal section of CT scan showing the vertical position of the station 10L lymph node which is usually one intercartilage space below the carina.*

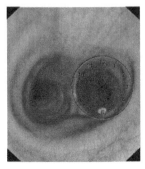

Fig. 6.9e *Bronchoscopic view of the station 10L lymph node which is in the 6 o'clock position about one intercartilage space below the carina in the left main bronchus.*

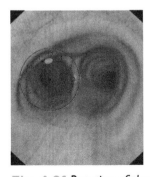

Fig. 6.9f *Rotation of the bronchoscope by 180° clockwise facilitates access of the station 10L lymph node.*

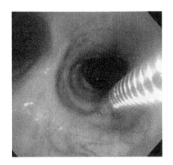

Fig. 6.9g *Bronchoscopic view of the needle inserted into a 10L lymph node with the scope rotated clockwise by 180°.*

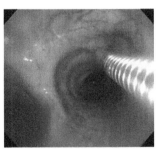

Fig. 6.9h *Bronchoscopic view of the needle inserted into a 10L lymph node in the 6 o'clock position with the scope in the neutral position.*

Station 11Rs: Right upper hilar lymph node (Fig. 6.10)

The station 11R includes the right upper and right lower hilar nodes. The right upper hilar node is located on the CT scan between the right upper lobe bronchus and the bronchus intermedius. On the CT cross-section it relates to the 9 o'clock position just below the origin of the bronchus intermedius. At bronchoscopy this relates to the anterior spur of the right upper lobe carina and the optimal approach is to insert the needle just below the spur of the upper lobe carina. When the patient is approached from the front, this is just below the origin of the bronchus intermedius in the 9–10 o'clock position. It is in the proximal portion of the bronchus intermedius.

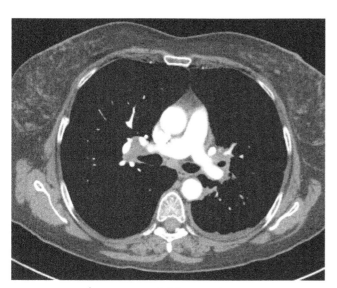

Fig. 6.10a *Cross-sectional CT scan of the thorax showing a station 11Rs (right upper hilar) lymph node.*

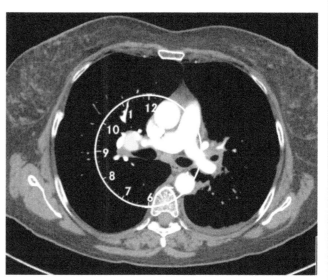

Fig. 6.10b *Cross-sectional CT scan with a superimposed clock face and a station 11Rs (right upper hilar) lymph node highlighted in yellow.*

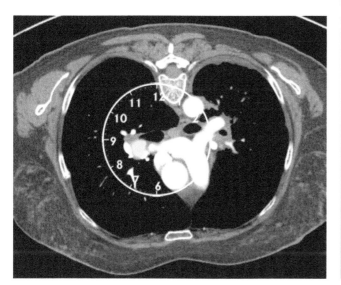

Fig. 6.10c *Cross-sectional CT scan of the thorax flipped on the horizontal axis. The station 11Rs (right upper hilar) lymph node is in the 9 o'clock position.*

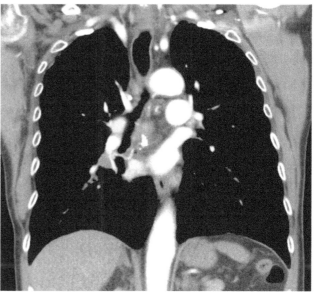

Fig. 6.10d *Coronal section of CT scan showing the vertical position of the station 11Rs (right upper hilar) lymph node, which is usually located at the right upper lobe carina.*

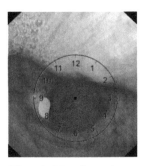

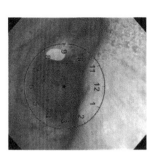

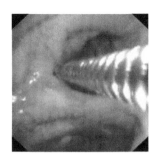

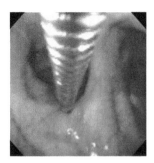

Fig. 6.10e *Bronchoscopic view of the station 11Rs (right upper hilar) lymph node which is in the 9 o'clock position in the anterior spur of the right upper lobe carina.*

Fig. 6.10f *Rotation of the bronchoscope by 90° clockwise facilitates access of the station 11Rs (right upper hilar) lymph node.*

Fig. 6.10g *Bronchoscopic view of the needle inserted into a station 11Rs (right upper hilar) lymph node with the scope rotated clockwise by 90°.*

Fig. 6.10h *Bronchoscopic view of the needle inserted into a station 11Rs (right upper hilar) lymph node in the 9 o'clock position with the scope in the neutral position.*

Station 11Ri: Right lower hilar lymph node (Fig. 6.11)

On the CT scan, the right lower hilar lymph node is located lateral to the bronchus intermedius in the 9 o'clock position at the level of the right middle lobe. At bronchoscopy the needle should be inserted in the distal part of the bronchus intermedius in the 9 o'clock position at the level of the right middle lobe origin. Access into this lymph node is also facilitated by rotation of the scope by 90°.

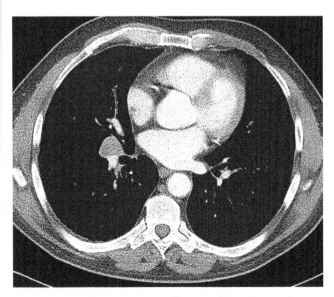

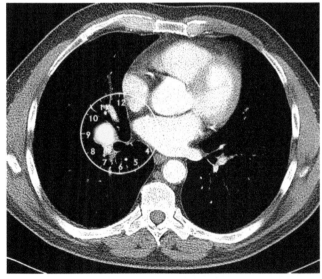

Fig. 6.11a *Cross-sectional CT scan of the thorax showing a station 11Ri (right lower hilar) lymph node.*

Fig. 6.11b *Cross-sectional CT scan with a superimposed clock face and a station 11Ri (right lower hilar) lymph node highlighted in yellow.*

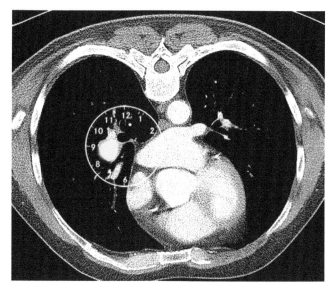

Fig. 6.11c *Cross-sectional CT scan of the thorax flipped on the horizontal axis. The station 11Ri (right lower hilar) lymph node is in the 9 o'clock position.*

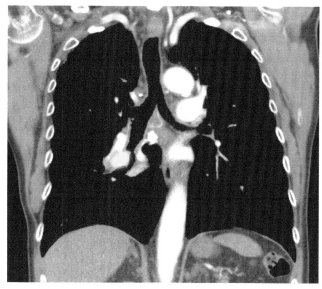

Fig. 6.11d *Coronal section of CT scan showing the vertical position of the station 11Ri (right lower hilar) lymph node, which is usually just higher than the right middle lobe origin.*

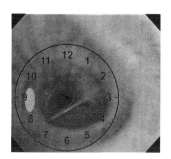

Fig. 6.11e *Bronchoscopic view of the station 11Ri (right lower hilar) lymph node which is in the 9 o'clock position in the bronchus intermedius just above the origin of the right middle lobe.*

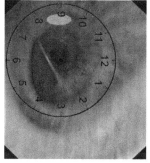

Fig. 6.11f *Rotation of the bronchoscope by 90° clockwise facilitates access of the station 11Ri (right lower hilar) lymph node.*

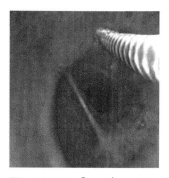

Fig. 6.11g *Bronchoscopic view of the needle inserted into a station 11Ri (right lower hilar) lymph node with the scope rotated clockwise by 90°.*

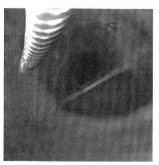

Fig. 6.11h *Bronchoscopic view of the needle inserted into a station 11Ri (right lower hilar) lymph node in the 9 o'clock position with the scope in the neutral position.*

Station 11L: Left hilar lymph node (Fig. 6.12)

The station 11L or left hilar lymph node is located at the bifurcation of the left main bronchus. It is accessed from the left lower lobe towards the upper lobe in the 6–7 o'clock position. Needle insertion is easier if the bronchoscope is rotated by 180° and the needle is inserted into the 12–1 o'clock position from the left lower lobe to the left upper lobe.

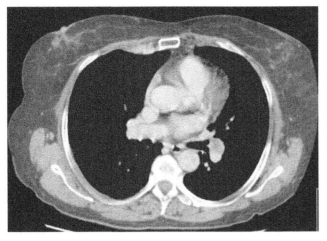

Fig. 6.12a *Cross-sectional CT scan of the thorax showing a station 11L lymph node.*

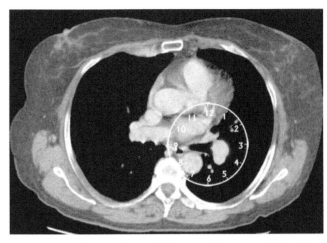

Fig. 6.12b *Cross-sectional CT scan with a superimposed clock face and a station 11L lymph node highlighted in yellow.*

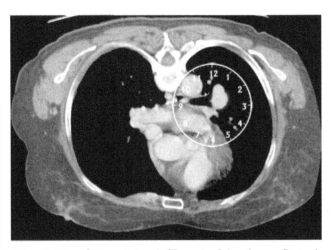

Fig. 6.12c *Cross-sectional CT scan of the thorax flipped on the horizontal axis. The 11L lymph node is in the 6–7 o'clock position when approached from the left lower lobe.*

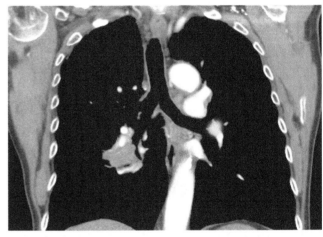

Fig. 6.12d *Coronal section of CT scan showing the vertical position of the station 11L lymph node which is usually at the level of the carina between the left upper and lower lobes.*

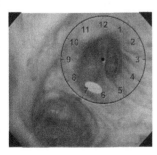

Fig. 6.12e *Bronchoscopic view of the station 11L lymph node which is in the 6–7 o'clock position when approached from the left lower lobe and about one intercartilage space below the left main bronchial carina.*

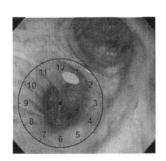

Fig. 6.12f *Rotation of the bronchoscope by 180° clockwise facilitates access of the station 11L lymph node and the lymph node is in the 12 to 1 o'clock position when approached from the left lower lobe and about one intercartilage space below the left main bronchial carina.*

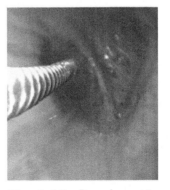

Fig. 6.12g *Bronchoscopic view of the needle inserted into an 11L lymph node with the scope rotated anticlockwise by 90°.*

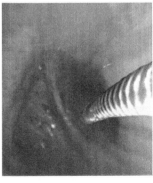

Fig. 6.12h *Bronchoscopic view of the needle inserted into an 11L lymph node in the 3 o'clock position with the scope in the neutral position.*

Transbronchial fine-needle aspiration (posterior approach)

Transbronchial fine-needle aspiration (TBNA) is a simple, cheap technique for sampling mediastinal nodes. Hilar lymph nodes, masses adjacent to the airways and submucosal disease may also be sampled with this technique. A variety of needles are available but the needle should be retractable with a length of between 13 and 15 mm and a gauge of between 18 and 22 (Fig. 7.1).

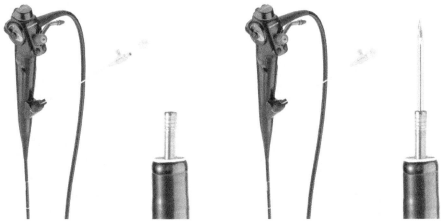

Fig 7.1a *Bronchoscope with transbronchial fine-needle aspiration needle: withdrawn into the sheath.*

Fig 7.1b *Bronchoscope with transbronchial fine-needle aspiration needle: extended out of the sheath.*

Planning/site selection

The computed tomography (CT) scan of the thorax should be examined prior to TBNA and the site of aspiration should be predetermined (Fig. 7.2a). The simplest approach is to relate the airway to a clock face and plan the position of target sites in this manner (Fig. 7.2b). The CT scan is obtained by imaging from the feet upwards (Fig. 7.2c), whereas at bronchoscopy the patient is approached from the head downwards (Fig. 7.2d). It is therefore important to account for these differences. For patients who are being approached from the posterior side, the simple trick is to flip the image in the vertical axis (Fig. 7.2e). The vertical position also needs to be determined and can be described in terms of cartilage spaces or rings above and below the carina (Fig. 7.2f). In some cases it may be necessary to relate the vertical position to the origin of the segmental bronchi. More detailed descriptions are given for the example lymph node stations in this chapter, but it should be emphasized that this is merely a guide and individual sites for aspiration are determined according to the patient's CT scan. Modern multi-planar reformatting of CTs and software modules with virtual bronchoscopy (Fig. 7.2g) and lymph node highlighting (Fig. 7.2h) may help to determine the site of needle aspiration.

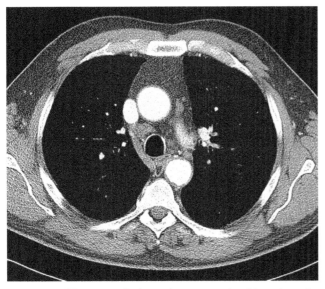

Fig 7.2a *CT scan with the right paratracheal lymph node present.*

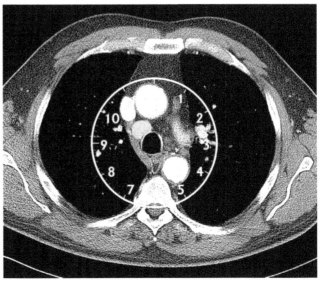

Fig 7.2b *CT scan with the right paratracheal lymph node highlighted in yellow and the clock face showing that the lymph node is in 10–11 o'clock position.*

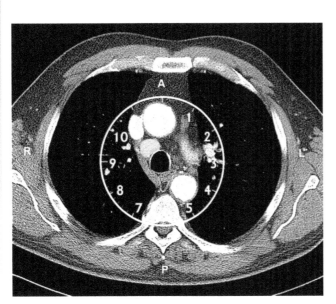

Fig 7.2c *Cross-sectional CT scan of the thorax; note the relative position of the anterior and posterior aspects of the patient.*

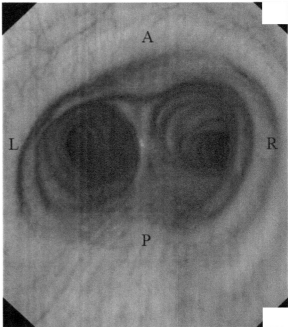

Fig 7.2d *Bronchoscopic view; note the relative position of the anterior and posterior aspects of the patient.*

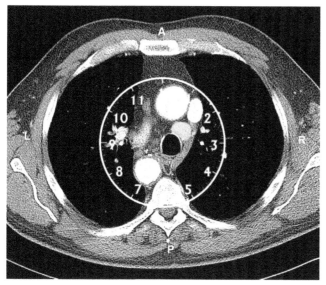

Fig 7.2e *Cross-sectional CT scan of the thorax flipped on the vertical axis so as to align the right and left aspects of the patient with the bronchoscopic view.*

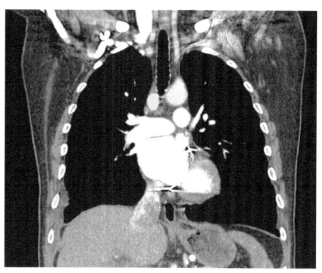

Fig 7.2f *Coronal CT reformat to help determine the vertical position of the lymph node in relation to the carina.*

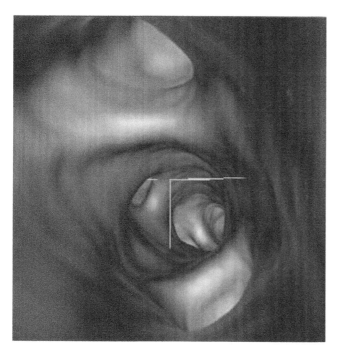

Fig 7.2g *Virtual bronchoscopy derived from CT scanning.*

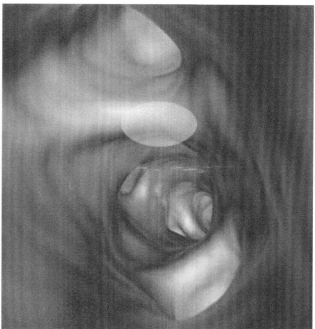

Fig 7.2h *Virtual bronchoscopy derived from CT scanning with lymph node highlighting.*

Technique

Transbronchial fine-needle aspiration should be performed first during the bronchoscopy and, in the case of mediastinal lymph node sampling, before inspection of the airways. Minimal use of suction should be employed in order to minimize the risk of aspirating cellular material from the distal airways, which may lead to false-positive results. These simple precautions virtually prevent any false-positive results. This is important in the staging of lung cancer where a false-positive result would upstage a patient and deny him or her potentially curative surgery. It is also important to sample the highest-stage lymph nodes first, e.g. N3 lymph nodes followed by N2 lymph nodes and finally N1 lymph nodes. The needle should be inserted through the instrument channel of the bronchoscope with the bronchoscope as straight as possible in the trachea. Any flexion or extension of the distal portion of the scope should be avoided until the hub of the needle is outside the bronchoscope. This is essential in order to minimize bronchoscope damage.

A number of techniques can be used to sample the lymph node:

- jabbing
- piggyback
- cough.

● Jabbing technique

This involves guiding the bronchoscope to the target area and then apposing the distal hub of the needle to the airway wall. The distal portion of the scope should be angulated to ensure that the needle penetrates through the airway as perpendicular as possible. There should be an angle of at least 45° between the airway wall and the needle (Fig. 7.3). The needle is then pushed through the airway wall and gently manipulated back and forth. At the same time, an assistant should apply suction at the

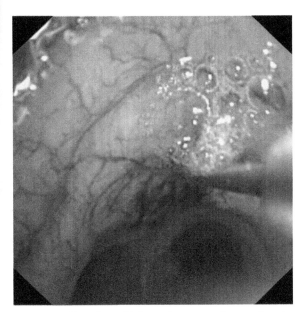

Fig. 7.3a *Transbronchial needle apposed on to the airway wall at an angle of a least 45° in the anterior carinal position.*

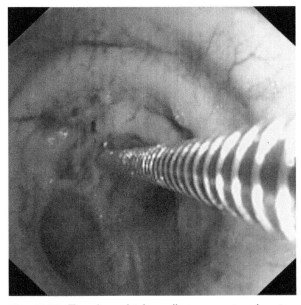

Fig. 7.3b *Transbronchial needle penetrating the airway wall in the anterior carinal position.*

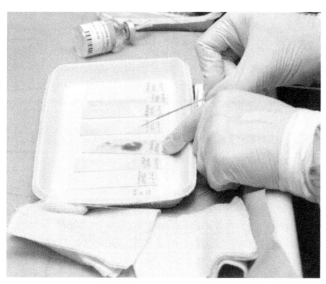

Fig. 7.3c *Cytology smears prepared by spraying aspirates on to the slides.*

proximal end of the TBNA needle with a 20 mL syringe. The samples collected are then smeared on to slides and sprayed with a fixative, or alternatively injected into saline or cytolyte solution, depending on the preference of the local site pathologist. Any tissue fragments or slivers obtained are placed in formalin and sent for histological analysis. The availability of rapid on-site cytological evaluation (ROSE) significantly reduces the time of the procedure and improves diagnostic yield.

In the absence of a ROSE, at least four needle passes are made at each target site when assessing patients with suspected lung cancer. The site with the highest possible lymph node stage should be sampled first, then moving progressively down to the lower site.

Piggyback method

With this method the needle is advanced, and once the hub is protruding through the distal end, the needle is fixed by pressing the insertion port of the bronchoscope with an index finger. This does cause the catheter to bend at this point and the technique is better reserved for single-use disposable needles. Once the needle is fixed into position, the scope and the needle can be moved in unison and pushed forward at the desired location until the needle penetrates the airway wall. The needle is moved back and forth with an assistant applying suction as described for the jabbing technique.

Cough technique

This method employs either of the above approaches in conjunction with a controlled cough to facilitate penetration of the needle through the airway wall. It relies on patient cooperation and may not always be successful.

Lymph node stations

It is possible to sample any of the lymph nodes that are adjacent to the airways using TBNA. The lymph node stations are described according to the new International Association for the Study of Lung Cancer (IASLC) classification.

● *Superior mediastinal lymph nodes: upper zone*

Station 4R: Lower right paratracheal lymph node (Fig. 7.4)

The right paratracheal lymph node is classically located in the right anterior aspect of the trachea. The exact position should be predetermined from the CT scan. Usually on the CT scan the right paratracheal lymph node is located in the 10–11 o'clock position if the anterior midline is considered to be 12 o'clock. However, one should note that the CT scans are obtained by looking at the patient from the feet upwards; but when patients undergo a bronchoscopy, the airways are viewed with the head downwards. When the patient is approached from the back with the patient supine, their right side is now at the 3 o'clock position and the left side at the 9 o'clock position. Hence, in this position the right paratracheal lymph node is actually positioned between the 1 and 2 o'clock position. The simplest way is to flip the CT scan on the vertical axis. The vertical position of the right paratracheal lymph node is about two to four intercartilage spaces above the carina.

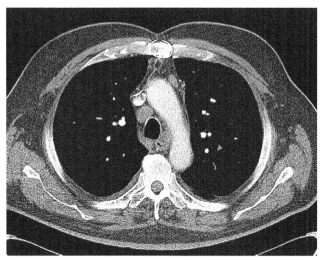

Fig. 7.4a *Cross-sectional CT scan of the thorax at the level of the aortic arch showing a station 4R lymph node.*

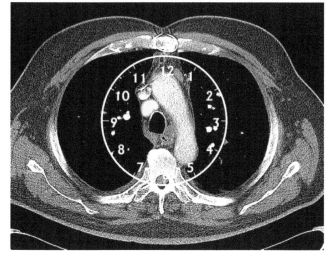

Fig. 7.4b *Cross-sectional CT scan with a superimposed clock face and a station 4R lymph node highlighted in yellow.*

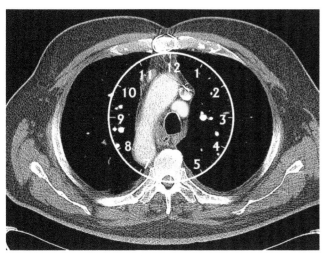

Fig. 7.4c *Cross-sectional CT scan of the thorax flipped on the vertical axis. The 4R lymph node is in the 1–2 o'clock position.*

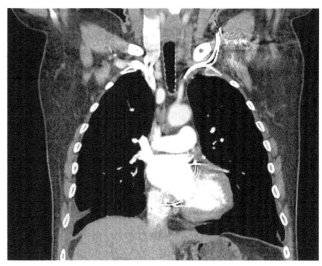

Fig. 7.4d *Coronal section of CT scan showing the vertical position of the lymph node, which is usually about two to four rings above the carina.*

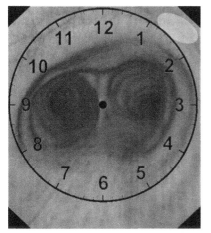

Fig. 7.4e *Bronchoscopic view of the station 4R lymph node which is in the 1–2 o'clock position about two to four intercartilage spaces above the carina.*

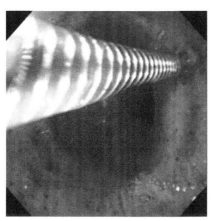

Fig. 7.4f *Bronchoscopic view of the needle inserted into a 4R lymph node in the 2 o'clock position.*

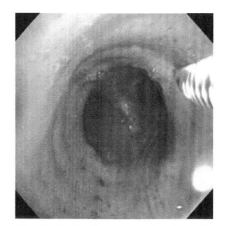

Fig. 7.4g *Further example of needle inserted into the 4R lymph node.*

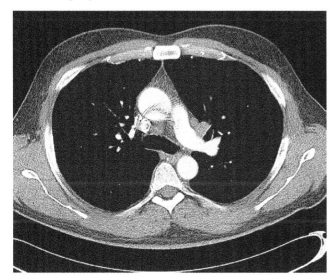

Fig. 7.4h *Cross-sectional CT scan of the thorax at the level of the carina showing an anterior carinal lymph node (station 4R lymph node).*

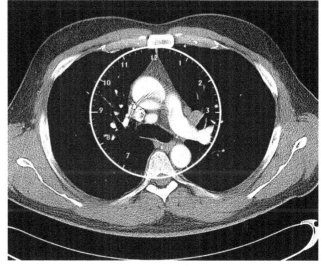

Fig. 7.4i *Cross-sectional CT scan of the thorax at the level of the carina with a superimposed clock face and highlighting an anterior carinal lymph node (station 4R lymph node).*

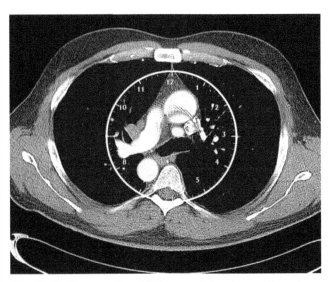

Fig. 7.4j *Cross-sectional CT scan of the thorax flipped on the vertical axis. The anterior carinal lymph node is in the 12–12.30 o'clock position.*

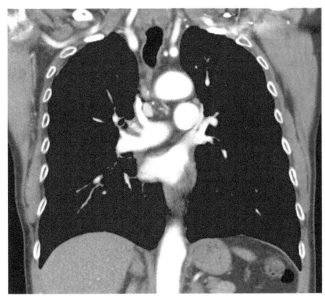

Fig. 7.4k *Coronal section of CT scan showing the vertical position of the lymph node, which is usually at the level of the carina.*

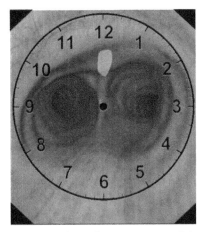

Fig. 7.4l *Bronchoscopic view of the anterior carinal (station 4R) lymph node which is in the 12 o'clock position at the level of the carina.*

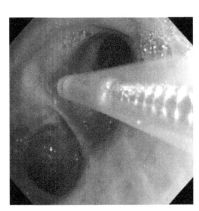

Fig. 7.4m *Bronchoscopic view of the needle inserted into the anterior carinal lymph node in the 12 o'clock position.*

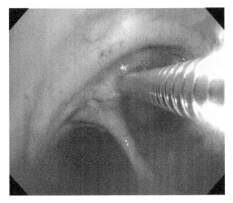

Fig. 7.4n *Bronchoscopic view of the needle inserted into the anterior carinal lymph node in the 12.30 o'clock position.*

As described in Chapter 5, the station 4R can extend anterior to the trachea through to the 2 o'clock position. Nodes located anterior to the trachea were previously described as anterior carinal lymph nodes. It is usually located in the 11.30–12 o'clock position on the CT scan. In patients being bronchoscoped from behind, this is the 12–12.30 position.

Station 4L: Lower left paratracheal lymph node (Fig. 7.5)

The left paratracheal lymph node is located on the left lateral position of the trachea at or above the level of the carina. On the CT scan the lymph node is located at the 3 o'clock position. When the patient is being approached from behind, at bronchoscopy the lymph node is located at the 9 o'clock position. The vertical position of the lymph node is at the level of the carina or one space above. In practice this lymph node is more easily accessed by rotating the bronchoscope 90° in a clockwise direction. Once the needle has penetrated the airway wall, the torsion on the bronchoscope can be relaxed and the needle moved back while the bronchoscope is in the neutral position (as in Fig. 7.5h).

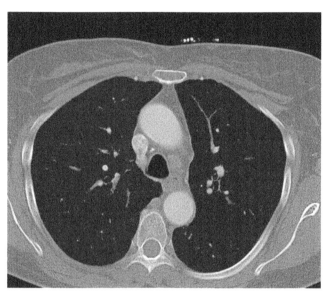

Fig. 7.5a *Cross-sectional CT scan of the thorax showing a station 4L lymph node.*

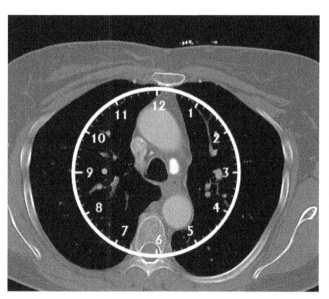

Fig. 7.5b *Cross-sectional CT scan with a superimposed clock face and a station 4L lymph node highlighted in yellow.*

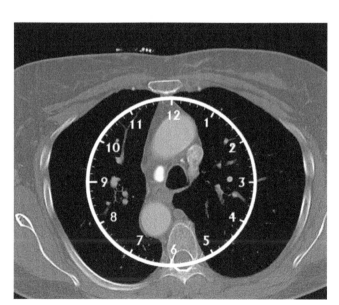

Fig. 7.5c *Cross-sectional CT scan of the thorax flipped on the vertical axis. The 4L lymph node is in the 9 o'clock position.*

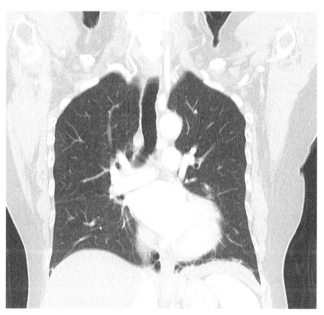

Fig. 7.5d *Coronal section of CT scan showing the vertical position of the station 4L lymph node which is usually at one intercartilage space above the carina.*

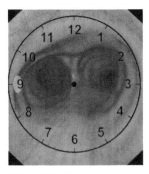

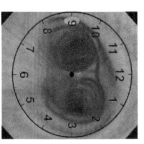

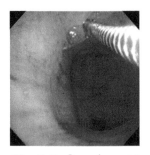

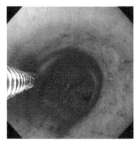

Fig. 7.5e *Bronchoscopic view of the station 4L lymph node, which is in the 9 o'clock position about one intercartilage space above the carina.*

Fig. 7.5f *Rotation of the bronchoscope by 90° clockwise facilitates access to the station 4L lymph node.*

Fig. 7.5g *Bronchoscopic view of the needle inserted into a 4L lymph node with the scope rotated clockwise by 90°.*

Fig. 7.5h *Bronchoscopic view of the needle inserted into a 4L lymph node in the 9 o'clock position with the scope in the neutral position.*

Station 3P: Posterior tracheal lymph node (Fig. 7.6)

The posterior carinal lymph node is located at the level of the carina on the posterior aspect of the trachea. On CT terms it can be considered to be in the 5.30–6 position. At bronchoscopy when the patient is approached from behind, the lymph nodes are now located at the 6–6.30 o'clock position. The forward angulation of the bronchoscope is greater in the anterior direction and therefore access for TBNA is improved by rotating the scope to 180° so that the lymph nodes are now anterior in the 11.30–12 o'clock position.

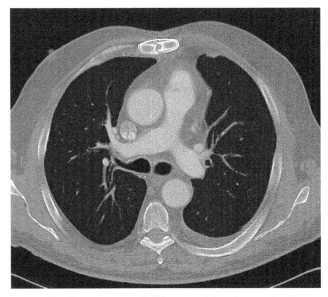

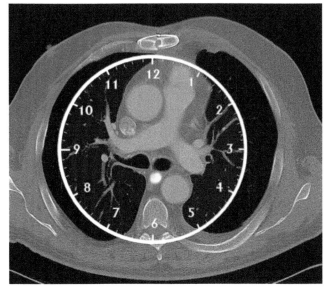

Fig. 7.6a *Cross-sectional CT scan of the thorax showing a station 3p lymph node.*

Fig. 7.6b *Cross-sectional CT scan with a superimposed clock face and a station 3p lymph node highlighted in yellow.*

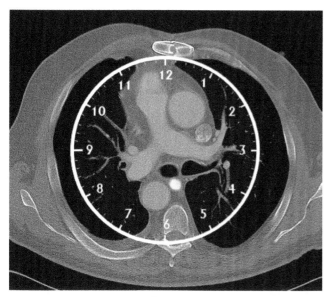

Fig. 7.6c *Cross-sectional CT scan of the thorax flipped on the vertical axis. The 3p lymph node is in the 6–6.30 o'clock position.*

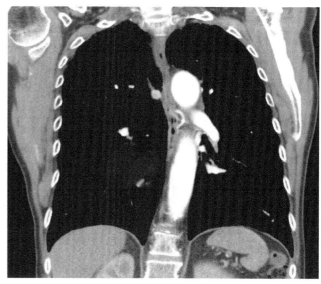

Fig. 7.6d *Coronal section of CT scan showing the vertical position of the station 3p lymph node which is usually at the level of the carina.*

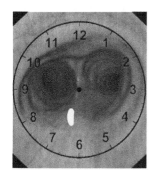

Fig. 7.6e *Bronchoscopic view of the station 3p lymph node which is in the 6–6.30 o'clock position about one intercartilage space above the carina.*

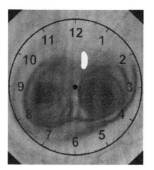

Fig. 7.6f *Rotation of the bronchoscope by 180° facilitates access to the station 3p lymph node.*

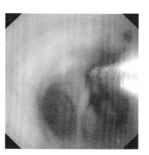

Fig. 7.6g *Bronchoscopic view of the needle inserted into a 3p lymph node with the scope rotated clockwise by 180°.*

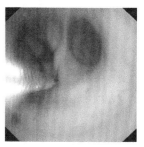

Fig. 7.6h *Bronchoscopic view of the needle inserted into a 3p lymph node in the 6 o'clock position with the scope in the neutral position.*

● Inferior mediastinal lymph nodes

Station 7: Subcarinal lymph node (Fig. 7.7)

The subcarinal lymph nodes are located just inferior to the carina. The carina is composed of three bundles of cartilage and ligament, and hence direct puncture through the carina tends to be unsuccessful. The subcarinal lymph nodes should be approached in the right main bronchus at one space below the carina. On the CT scan this translates to the 3 o'clock position and it is at the 9 o'clock position (medially in the right main bronchus one space below the carina) when the patient is being bronchoscoped from behind.

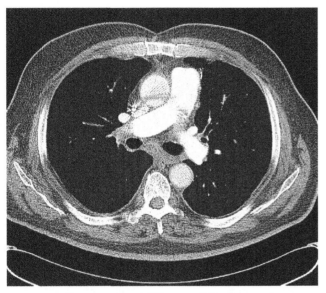

Fig. 7.7a *Cross-sectional CT scan of the thorax showing a station 7 lymph node.*

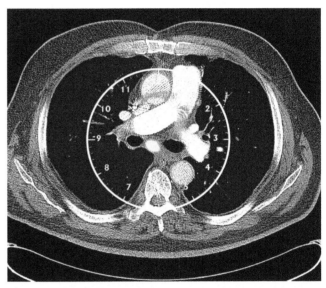

Fig. 7.7b *Cross-sectional CT scan with a superimposed clock face and a station 7 lymph node highlighted in yellow.*

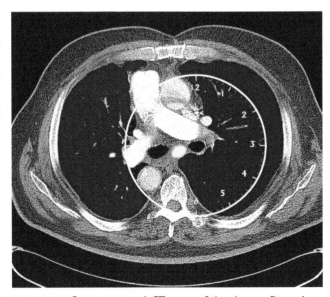

Fig. 7.7c *Cross-sectional CT scan of the thorax flipped on the vertical axis. The station 7 lymph node is in the 9 o'clock position.*

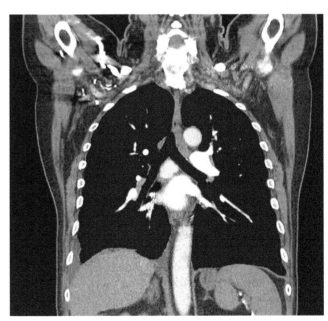

Fig. 7.7d *Coronal section of CT scan showing the vertical position of the station 4L lymph node, which is usually at one intercartilage space above the carina.*

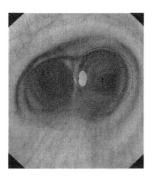

Fig. 7.7e *Bronchoscopic view of the station 7 lymph node which is in the 9 o'clock position one intercartilage space below the carina in the right main bronchus.*

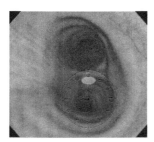

Fig. 7.7f *Rotation of the bronchoscope 90° clockwise facilitates access to the station 7 lymph node.*

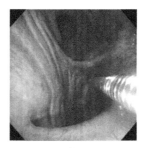

Fig. 7.7g *Bronchoscopic view of the needle inserted into a station 7 lymph node with the scope rotated 90° clockwise.*

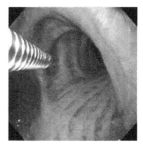

Fig. 7.7h *Bronchoscopic view of the needle inserted into a station 7 lymph node in the 9 o'clock position with the scope in the neutral position.*

Hilar zone lymph nodes

Station 10R: Right main bronchial lymph node (Fig. 7.8)

The right main bronchial node is located anterior to the right main bronchus about one intercartilage space below the carina at the 12 o'clock position on the CT scan. When the patient is being approached from behind, the lymph node is also located in the 12 o'clock position in the right main bronchus one space below the carina.

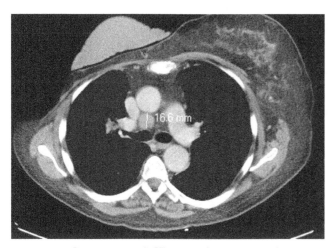

Fig. 7.8a *Cross-sectional CT scan of the thorax showing a station 10R lymph node.*

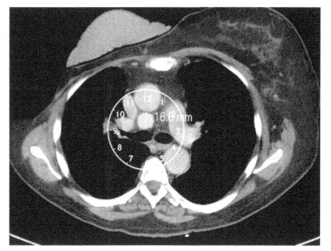

Fig. 7.8b *Cross-sectional CT scan with a superimposed clock face and a station 10R lymph node highlighted in yellow.*

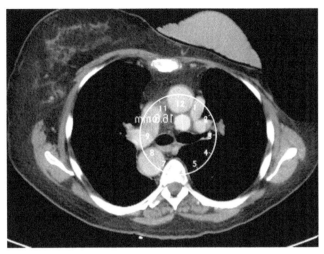

Fig. 7.8c *Cross-sectional CT scan of the thorax flipped on the vertical axis. The 10R lymph node is in the 12 o'clock position in the right main bronchus.*

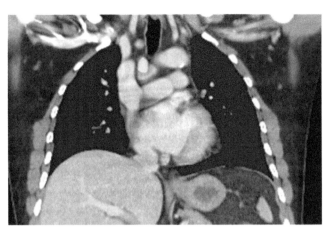

Fig. 7.8d *Coronal section of CT scan showing the vertical position of the station 10R lymph node which is usually one intercartilage space below the carina in the right main bronchus.*

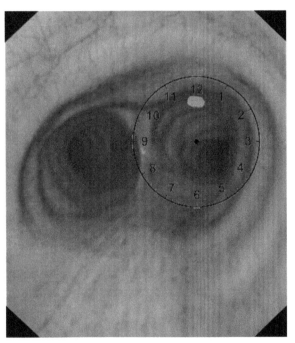

Fig. 7.8e *Bronchoscopic view of the station 10R lymph node which is in the 12 o'clock position about one intercartilage space below the carina in the right main bronchus.*

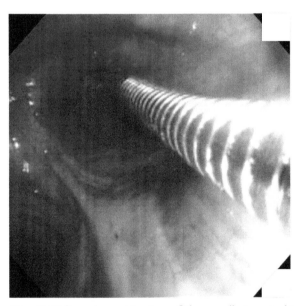

Fig. 7.8f *Bronchoscopic view of the needle inserted into a 10R lymph node.*

Station 10L: Left main bronchial lymph node (Fig. 7.9)

The left main bronchial lymph node is located on the anterior aspect of the left main bronchus approximately one interspace below the carina in the 12 o'clock position. This is naturally the position in which the lymph node is located when the patient is being bronchoscoped from behind.

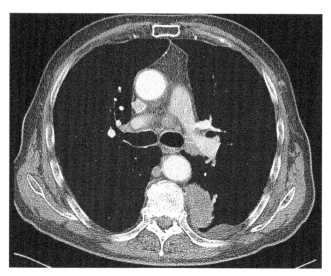

Fig. 7.9a *Cross-sectional CT scan of the thorax showing a station 10L lymph node.*

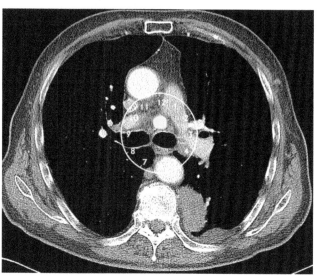

Fig. 7.9b *Cross sectional CT scan with a superimposed clock face and a station 10L lymph node highlighted in yellow in the 12 o'clock position.*

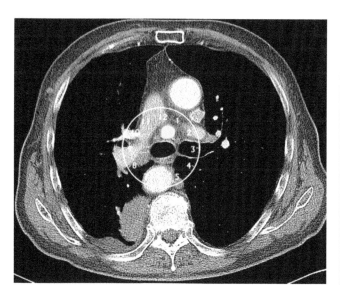

Fig. 7.9c *Cross-sectional CT scan of the thorax flipped on the vertical axis. The 10L lymph node is in the 12 o'clock position.*

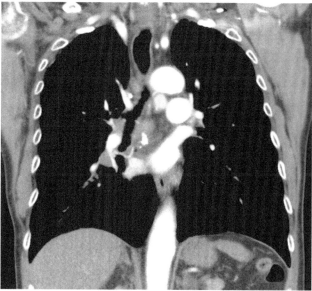

Fig. 7.9d *Coronal section of CT scan showing the vertical position of the station 10L lymph node which is usually one intercartilage space below the carina.*

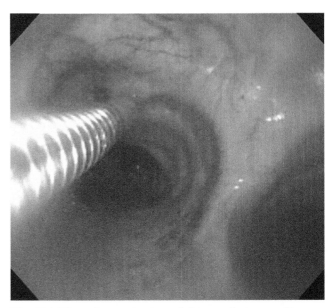

Fig. 7.9e *Bronchoscopic view of the station 10L lymph node which is in the 12 o'clock position about one intercartilage space below the carina in the left main bronchus.*

Fig. 7.9f *Bronchoscopic view of the needle inserted into a 10L lymph node.*

Station 11Rs: Right upper hilar lymph node (Fig. 7.10)

The right upper hilar node is located on the CT scan between the right upper lobe bronchus and the bronchus intermedius. On the CT cross-section it relates to the 9 o'clock position just below the origin of the bronchus intermedius. At bronchoscopy this relates to the anterior spur of the right upper lobe carina and the optimal approach is to insert the needle just below the spur of the upper lobe carina. When the patient is approached from behind, the right hilar node is located at the right side towards the 2–3 o'clock position in the anterior spur of the right upper lobe carina. It is in the proximal portion of the bronchus intermedius.

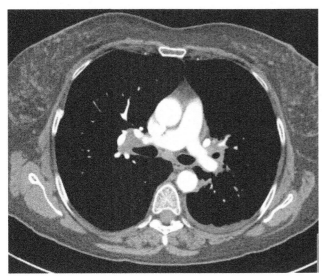

Fig. 7.10a *Cross-sectional CT scan of the thorax showing a station 11Rs (right upper hilar) lymph node.*

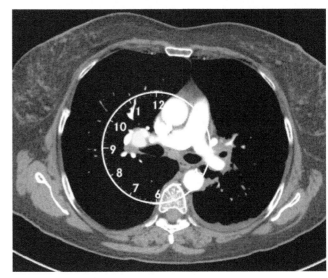

Fig. 7.10b *Cross-sectional CT scan with a superimposed clock face and a station 11Rs (right upper hilar) lymph node highlighted in yellow.*

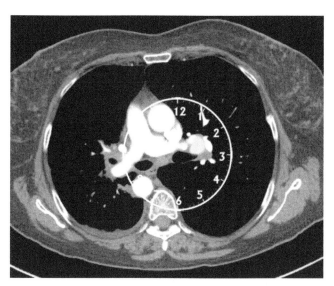

Fig. 7.10c *Cross-sectional CT scan of the thorax flipped on the vertical axis. The station 11Rs (right upper hilar) lymph node is in the 2–3 o'clock position.*

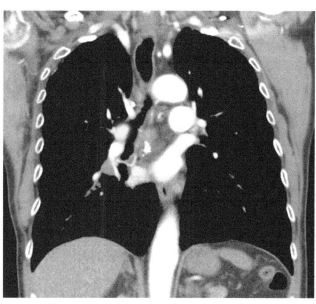

Fig. 7.10d *Coronal section of CT scan showing the vertical position of the station 11Rs (right upper hilar) lymph node, which is usually located at the right upper lobe carina.*

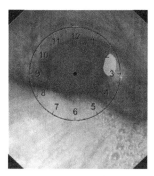

Fig. 7.10e *Bronchoscopic view of the station 11Rs (right upper hilar) lymph node which is in the 2–3 o'clock position in the anterior spur of the right upper lobe carina.*

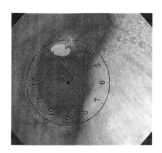

Fig. 7.10f *Rotation of the bronchoscope by 90° anticlockwise facilitates access to the station 11Rs (right upper hilar) lymph node.*

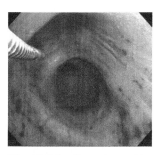

Fig. 7.10g *Bronchoscopic view of the needle inserted into a station 11Rs (right upper hilar) lymph node with the scope rotated 90° anticlockwise.*

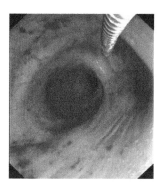

Fig. 7.10h *Bronchoscopic view of the needle inserted into a station 11Rs (right upper hilar) lymph node in the 2–3 o'clock position with the scope in the neutral position.*

Station 11Ri: Right lower hilar lymph node (Fig. 7.11)

On the CT scan the right lower hilar lymph node is located lateral to the bronchus intermedius in the 9 o'clock position at the level of the right middle lobe. At bronchoscopy the needle should be inserted in the 3 o'clock position in the distal aspect of the bronchus intermedius at the level of the right middle lobe origin.

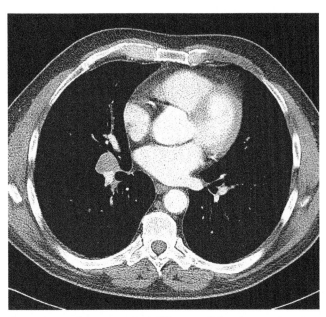

Fig. 7.11a *Cross-sectional CT scan of the thorax showing a station 11Ri (right lower hilar) lymph node.*

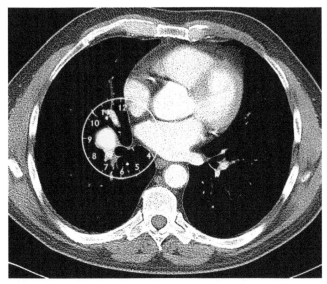

Fig. 7.11b *Cross-sectional CT scan with a superimposed clock face and a station 11Ri (right lower hilar) lymph node highlighted in yellow.*

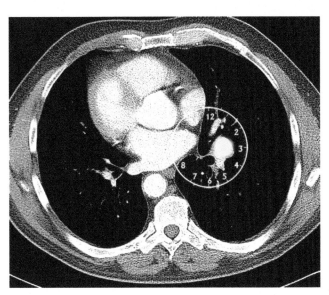

Fig. 7.11c *Cross-sectional CT scan of the thorax flipped on the vertical axis. The station 11Ri (right lower hilar) lymph node is in the 3 o'clock position.*

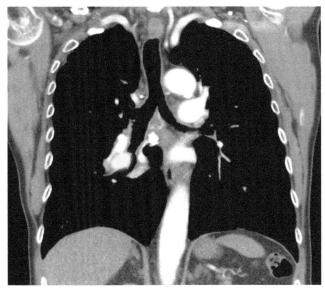

Fig. 7.11d *Coronal section of CT scan showing the vertical position of the station 11Ri (right lower hilar) lymph node, which is usually just higher than the right middle lobe origin.*

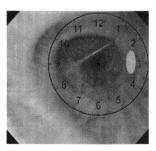

Fig. 7.11e *Bronchoscopic view of the station 11Ri (right lower hilar) lymph node, which is in the 3 o'clock position in the bronchus intermedius just above the origin of the right middle lobe.*

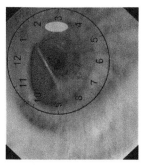

Fig. 7.11f *Rotation of the bronchoscope 90° anticlockwise facilitates access to the station 11Ri (right lower hilar) lymph node.*

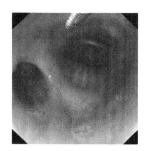

Fig. 7.11g *Bronchoscopic view of the needle inserted into a station 11Ri (right lower hilar) lymph node with the scope rotated 90° anticlockwise.*

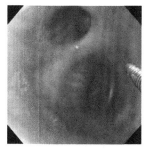

Fig. 7.11h *Bronchoscopic view of the needle inserted into a station 11Ri (right lower hilar) lymph node in the 3 o'clock position with the scope in the neutral position.*

Station 11L: Left hilar lymph node (Fig. 7.12)

The station 11L or left hilar lymph node is located at the bifurcation of the left main bronchus. It is accessed from the left lower lobe towards the upper lobe. The needle is inserted into the 11–12 o'clock position from the left lower to the left upper lobe.

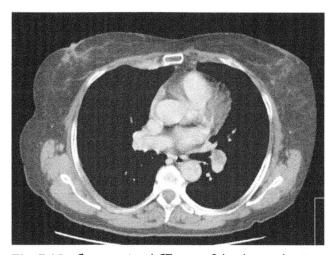

Fig. 7.12a *Cross-sectional CT scan of the thorax showing a station 11L lymph node.*

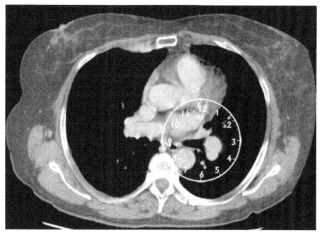

Fig. 7.12b *Cross-sectional CT scan with a superimposed clock face and a station 11L lymph node highlighted in yellow.*

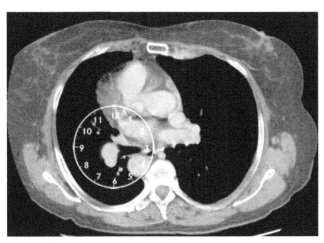

Fig. 7.12c *Cross-sectional CT scan of the thorax flipped on the horizontal axis. The 11L lymph node is in the 11–12 o'clock position.*

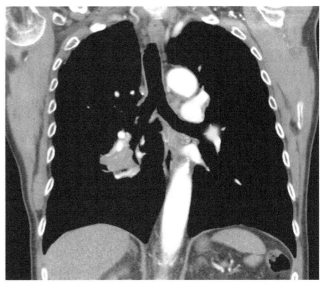

Fig. 7.12d *Coronal section of CT scan showing the vertical position of the station 11L lymph node, which is usually at level of the carina between the left upper and lower lobe.*

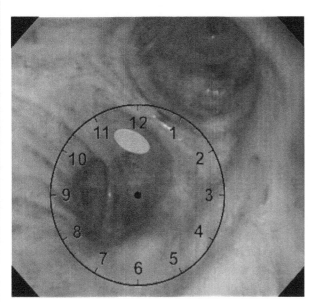

Fig. 7.12e *Bronchoscopic view of the station 11L lymph node which is in the 11–12 o'clock position about one intercartilage space above the carina.*

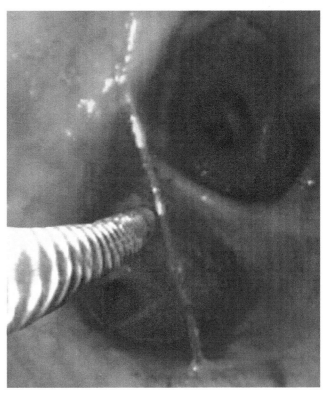

Fig. 7.12f *Bronchoscopic view of the needle inserted into an 11L lymph node in the 11–12 o'clock position.*

Endobronchial ultrasound bronchoscopy

Endobronchial ultrasound is usually performed using the oral approach with the patient lying supine and approached from behind. The current Olympus ultrasound bronchoscope has an offset viewing chip (Fig. 8.1). Hence it does not have a direct end-on view as in most bronchoscopes, with images offset in the upward direction of 30°. Hence a little practice is required to learn how to manipulate the bronchoscope, especially during the intubation phase.

The ultrasound image obtained can be improved by applying a water-filled balloon to the ultrasound transducer. This can be attached onto the distal end of the endobronchial ultrasound bronchoscope with a specific applicator. This water-filled balloon improves the acoustic contact but air bubbles within it may cause some artefacts.

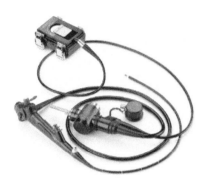

Fig. 8.1a *Endobronchial ultrasound bronchoscope.*

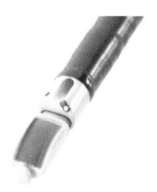

Fig. 8.1b *Distal tip of the endobronchial ultrasound bronchoscope with offset video chip.*

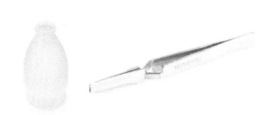

Fig. 8.1c *Balloon and applicator.*

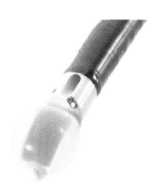

Fig. 8.1d *Distal view of the endobronchial ultrasound bronchoscope with water-filled balloon in place.*

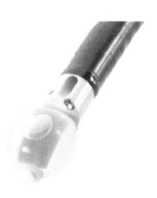

Fig. 8.1e *Distal view with air bubble visible within the water-filled balloon.*

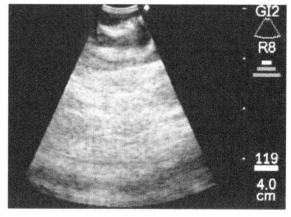

Fig. 8.1f *Artefact on ultrasound image due to air bubbles within the water-filled balloon.*

Intubation

During intubation the ideal view obtained of the cords is such that only the top of the vocal cords are in view and the cuneiform and corniculate tubercles are not visible. To obtain a full view of the cords, the scope needs to be angulated down (thumb up) (Fig. 8.2). However, the scope should not be advanced forward in this angulated position. The scope would simply meet resistance against the epiglottis in this position. The cords are prepared for intubation in the standard manner with the application of two to three aliquots of 1 mL of 2 per cent lidocaine. Further aliquots of lidocaine are applied to the trachea and main bronchus after intubation. The image obtained with the ultrasound bronchoscope is intended for intubation orientation within the airway. Although some diagnostic information is obtained, we would recommend using a conventional bronchoscope for these purposes and then use the ultrasound bronchoscope for mediastinal sampling.

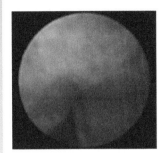 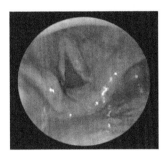 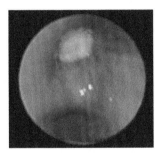 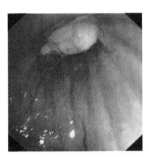

Fig. 8.2a *Bronchoscopic image of the vocal cords: with the scope straight.*

Fig. 8.2b *Bronchoscopic image of the vocal cords: with the scope angled down.*

Fig. 8.2c *Bronchoscopic image: with endobronchial ultrasound bronchoscope.*

Fig. 8.2d *Bronchoscopic image: with video bronchoscope.*

Examination approach

Our approach is to systematically examine all the lymph node stations. Additional areas which have been identified on a positron emission tomography (PET) or computed tomography (CT) scan should also be carefully examined. We would recommend first identifying the aortic arch which is located at the mid-trachea level on the left lateral wall of the trachea (Fig. 8.3).

Above the aortic arch are station 2 lymph nodes, and any paratracheal lymph nodes identified below the aortic arch are station 4 lymph nodes. So after identifying the aortic arch, the scope should be gently applied to the trachea wall and the more proximal trachea examined on both sides up to the subglottic level to check if any station 2 lymph nodes are visible. The bronchoscope is then rotated by about 150°–180° clockwise and the right paratracheal area (station 2R) examined. The scope is moved gently down until the brachiocephalic vein is visible. This denotes the lower limit of station 2R and any nodes below this area are station 4 lymph nodes.

During examination of the right paratracheal area (station 4R), the superior vena cava and the azygos vein should be identified. The lower limit of station 4R is denoted by the azygos vein. The scope is then moved anteriorly just at the level of the carina and the pulmonary trunk and the anterior carinal lymph nodes (station 4R) are examined. The scope is then further rotated anticlockwise towards the left lateral wall of the trachea at the level of the carina. First the ascending aorta is visualized and subsequently the left paratracheal lymph node area (station 4L) and then the pulmonary artery.

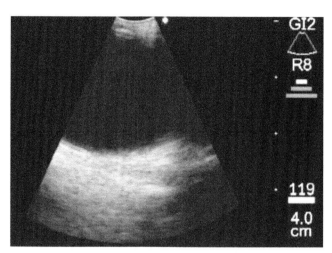

Fig. 8.3a *Ultrasound appearance of the aortic arch.*

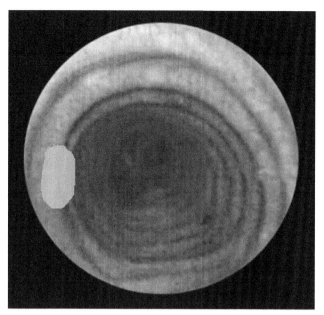

Fig. 8.3b *Bronchoscopic view of the trachea with the left lateral wall marked corresponding to the aortic arch.*

The scope is also run along the length of the posterior wall of the trachea to look for station 3p lymph nodes. The scope is then manoeuvred on to the medial aspect of the right main bronchus to examine the subcarinal lymph nodes (station 7).

The endobronchial scope is rotated by 90° clockwise in the right main bronchus so that it is facing the 12 o'clock position to examine the right hilar lymph nodes (station 10R). Following this, the scope is moved to the proximal aspect of the bronchus intermedius and the carina between the right upper lobe and the bronchus intermedius is examined. The right superior hilar nodes (station 11Rs) are located in this position. The bronchoscope is then rotated anticlockwise by 150° to examine the subcarinal lymph nodes (station 7), extending down to the distal margin of the bronchus intermedius. At the level of the right middle lobe the scope is again rotated 150° clockwise on to the lateral aspect of the bronchus intermedius, where the right inferior hilar (station 11Ri) is located.

The scope is then retracted back to the carina and the left side examined. Clockwise rotation by 90° and examination of the medial aspect of the left main bronchus allow station 7 to be examined from the left side. The scope can then be rotated back 90° anticlockwise to evaluate the left hilar lymph nodes (station 10L). Finally, the scope is applied to the carina between the left lower and upper lobe divisions. The left interlobar lymph node station (11L) is located at this site.

With endobronchial ultrasound, a key skill to acquire is navigation using ultrasound images. The anatomical landmarks should be used while learning the ultrasound anatomy. The combination of the endobronchial landmarks, location of blood vessels and ultrasound images should allow accurate characterization of the lymph node location and assignment to a specific lymph node station. With this systematic approach, all the lymph node locations adjacent to the endobronchial tree can be evaluated for accurate staging. The size and location of all the lymph nodes should be recorded. Any lymph nodes > 5 mm in size or with abnormal features (more rounded appearance, loss of large central blood vessels) should be sampled.

Lymph node stations

It is possible to sample any of the lymph nodes that are adjacent to the airways using transbronchial fine needle aspiration(TBNA). The lymph nodes stations are described according to the new International Association for the Study of Lung Cancer classification.

● *Superior mediastinal lymph nodes: upper zone*

Station 2R: Higher right paratracheal lymph node (Fig. 8.4)
The upper margin of station 2R is difficult to define at endobronchial ultrasound but is primarily at the level of the clavicle. The lower border is defined by the inferior aspect of the left brachiocephalic vein crossing the trachea. Anterolateral in this area, the right subclavian artery and right common carotid artery are visible on endobronchial ultrasound. More anterior to these blood vessels are the right brachiocephalic vein and the right external jugular vein. The endobronchial position is difficult to estimate accurately but is about one-third of the distance of the trachea from the vocal cords.

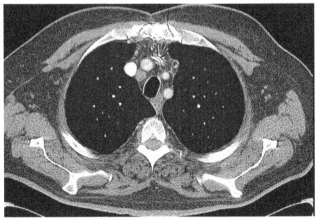

Fig. 8.4a *Cross-sectional CT scan of the thorax showing a station 2R lymph node.*

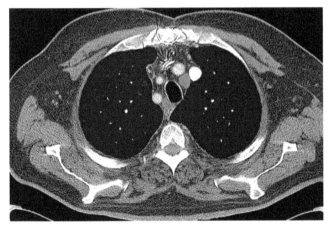

Fig. 8.4b *Cross-sectional CT scan flipped left to right with the station 2R lymph node highlighted in blue.*

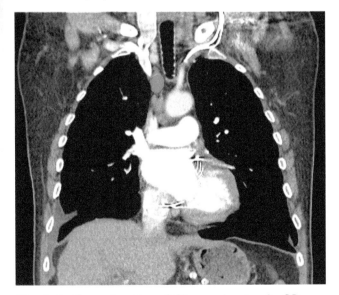

Fig. 8.4c *Coronal section of CT scan showing the 2R lymph node. Note that the node is above the level of the brachiocephalic vein crossing the trachea.*

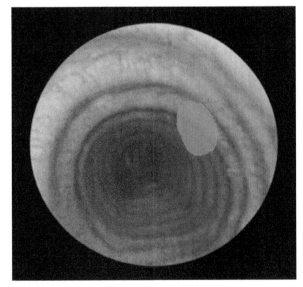

Fig. 8.4d *Bronchoscopic view of where the ultrasound probe should be placed to view the station 2R lymph nodes highlighted.*

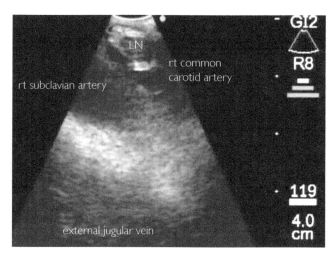

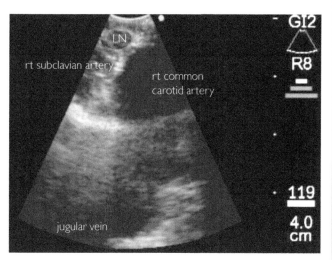

Fig. 8.4e Ultrasound image of the station 2R lymph node in a central position with the right common carotid artery superior to the node and the right subclavian artery inferior.

Fig. 8.4f Ultrasound image of the station 2R lymph node and the right common carotid artery more superior.

Station 2L: Higher left paratracheal lymph node (Fig. 8.5)

The upper border of station 2L is defined again by the clavicle and hence is difficult to define at endobronchial ultrasound. The lower border is determined by the aortic arch. On the left anterolateral aspects the common carotid and the left jugular vein are visible.

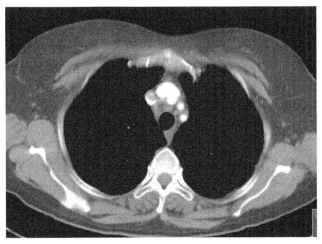

Fig. 8.5a *Cross-sectional CT scan of the thorax showing a station 2L lymph node.*

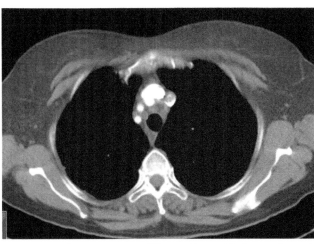

Fig. 8.5b *Cross-sectional CT scan flipped left to right with the station 2L lymph node highlighted in blue.*

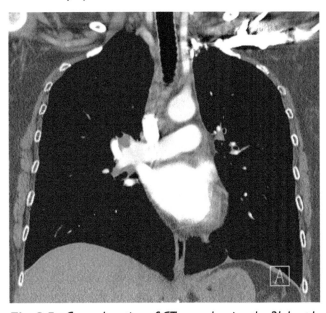

Fig. 8.5c *Coronal section of CT scan showing the 2L lymph node. Note the node is above the level of the aortic arch.*

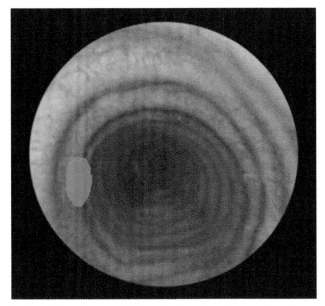

Fig. 8.5d *Bronchoscopic view of where the ultrasound probe should be placed to view the station 2L lymph nodes highlighted.*

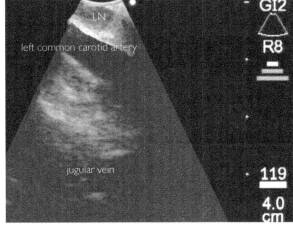

Fig. 8.5e *Ultrasound image of the station 2L lymph node.*

Station 3A: Anterior prevascular lymph node (Fig. 8.6)

The upper border is demarcated by the clavicle and the lower border by the carina, which is visible on the endobronchial image. These nodes are usually located anterior to the great vessels, i.e. the left common carotid and subclavian artery, and hence cannot be sampled by endobronchial ultrasound.

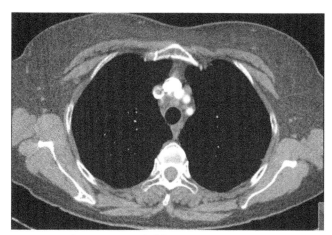

Fig. 8.6a *Cross-sectional CT scan of the thorax showing a station 3a lymph node.*

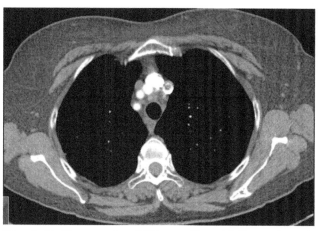

Fig. 8.6b *Cross-sectional CT scan flipped left to right with the station 3a lymph node highlighted.*

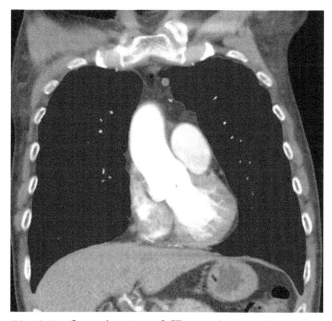

Fig. 8.6c *Coronal section of CT scan showing the station 3a lymph node.*

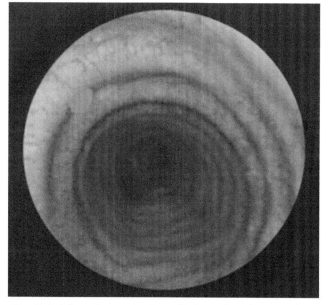

Fig. 8.6d *Bronchoscopic view of where the ultrasound probe should be placed to view the station 3a lymph nodes highlighted.*

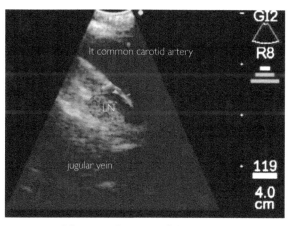

Fig. 8.6e *Ultrasound image of the station 3a lymph node.*

Station 3P: Posterior tracheal lymph node (Fig. 8.7)

The upper border is at the level of the clavicle and the lower border is at the carina, which can be confirmed by the bronchoscopic image. These nodes are located on the posterior aspect of the trachea.

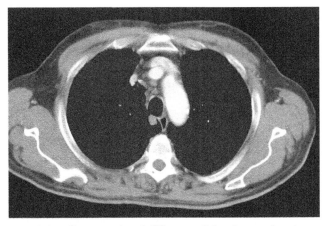

Fig. 8.7a *Cross-sectional CT scan of the thorax showing a station 3p lymph node.*

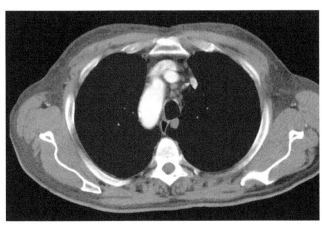

Fig. 8.7b *Cross-sectional CT scan flipped left to right with the station 3p lymph node highlighted.*

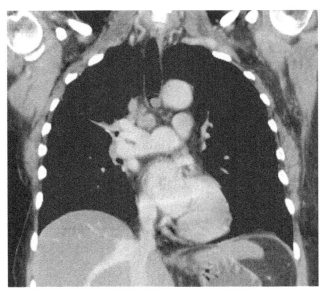

Fig. 8.7c *Coronal section of CT scan showing the station 3p lymph node.*

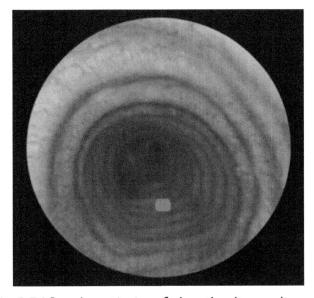

Fig. 8.7d *Bronchoscopic view of where the ultrasound probe should be placed to view the station 3p lymph nodes highlighted.*

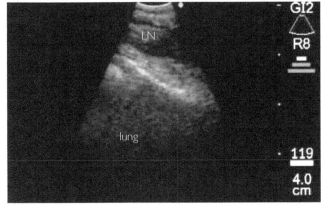

Fig. 8.7e *Ultrasound image of the station 3p lymph node.*

Station 4R: Lower right paratracheal lymph node (Fig. 8.8)

The upper border is identified on endobronchial ultrasound as the inferior margin of the brachiocephalic vein crossing the trachea. The lower border is defined by the azygos vein, which should be identified at ultrasound.

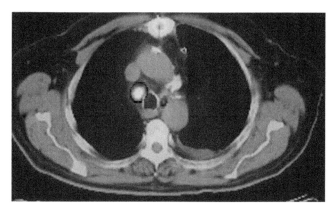

Fig. 8.8a *Cross-sectional PET-CT scan of the thorax showing an active station 4R lymph node.*

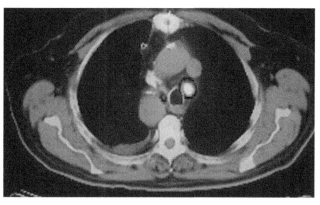

Fig. 8.8b *Cross-sectional PET-CT scan flipped left to right with the active station 4R lymph node.*

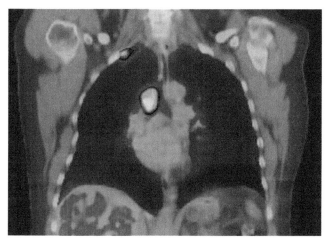

Fig. 8.8c *Coronal section of PET-CT scan showing the 4R lymph node.*

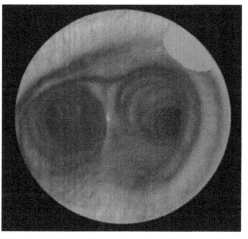

Fig. 8.8d *Bronchoscopic view of where the ultrasound probe should be placed to view the station 4R lymph nodes highlighted.*

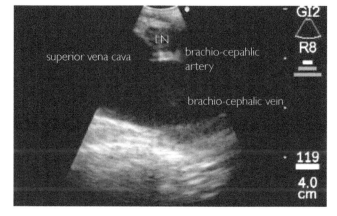

Fig. 8.8e *Ultrasound image of the station 4R lymph node with the brachiocephalic vein demarcating the border between stations 4R and 2R.*

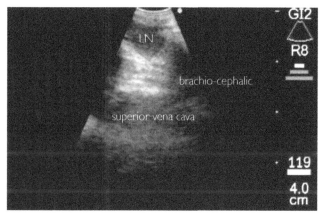

Fig. 8.8f *Ultrasound image of the station 4R lymph node.*

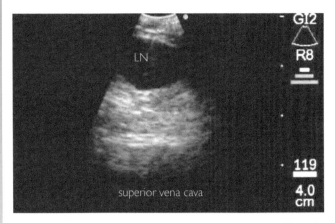

Fig. 8.8g *Ultrasound image of the station 4R lymph node with the superior vena cava more distal to the lymph node.*

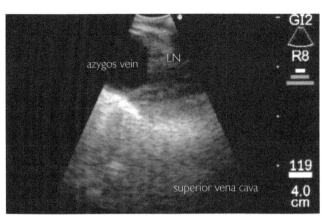

Fig. 8.8h *Ultrasound image of the station 4R lymph node with the azygos vein demarcating the border between station 4R and 10R lymph nodes.*

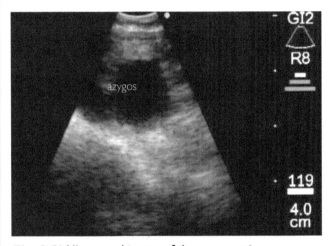

Fig. 8.8i *Ultrasound image of the azygos vein.*

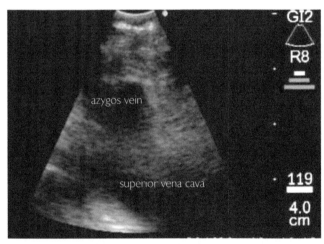

Fig. 8.8j *Ultrasound image of the azygos vein at a lower level with the superior vena cava visible distally.*

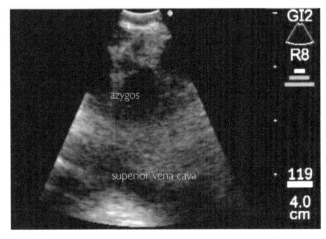

Fig. 8.8k *Ultrasound image of the azygos vein a few mm further distal.*

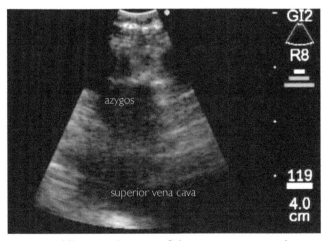

Fig. 8.8l *Ultrasound image of the azygos vein at a lower level draining into the superior vena cava.*

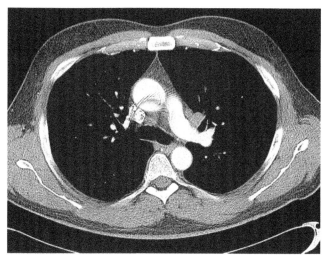

Fig. 8.8m *Further example of cross-sectional CT scan of the thorax showing a station 4R lymph node (anterior carinal lymph node).*

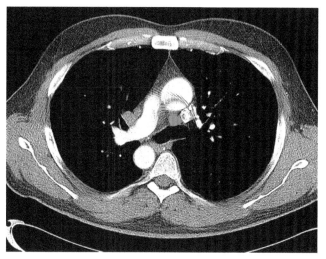

Fig. 8.8n *Cross-sectional CT scan flipped left to right with the station 4R (anterior carinal) lymph node highlighted.*

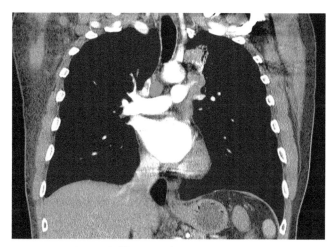

Fig. 8.8o *Coronal CT scan of the thorax showing an anterior carinal lymph node (station 4R lymph node).*

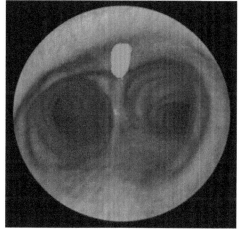

Fig. 8.8p *Bronchoscopic view of where the ultrasound probe should be placed to view the station 4R (anterior carinal node) lymph nodes highlighted.*

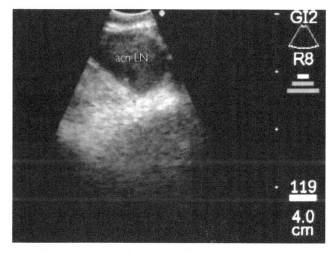

Fig. 8.8q *Ultrasound image of the station 4R (anterior carinal, acn) lymph node.*

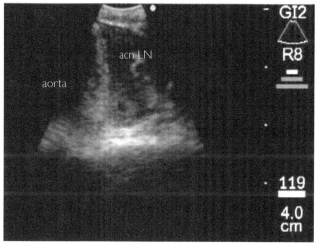

Fig. 8.8r *Ultrasound image of the station 4R (anterior carinal, acn) lymph node with the aorta visible just inferiorly.*

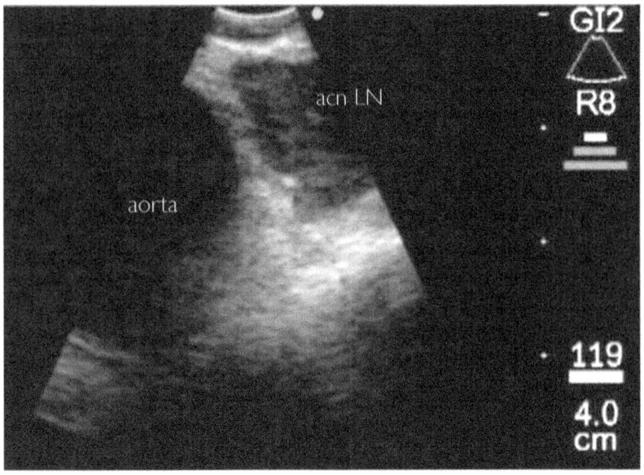

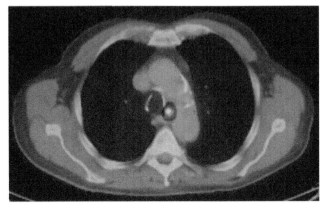

Fig. 8.8s *Ultrasound image of the station 4R (anterior carinal, acn) lymph node with a greater aspect of the aorta visible.*

The 4R lymph node is located anterolateral to the trachea, up to the left lateral border of the trachea. In the classical right paratracheal position, the superior vena cava is visible peripheral to the lymph node. As you move anteriorly towards the carina, the ascending aorta also becomes visible.

Station 4L: Lower left paratracheal lymph node (Fig. 8.9)
The location of the lymph node is between the ascending aorta and the pulmonary trunk. The upper border is defined by the aortic arch and the lower border by the pulmonary artery. The classical image visible at ultrasound consists of the lymph node identified in between the aorta which is on the right of the image and the pulmonary artery on the left of the image. The bronchoscopic location of this station is the left lateral aspect of the trachea at the level of the carina or one space above the carina.

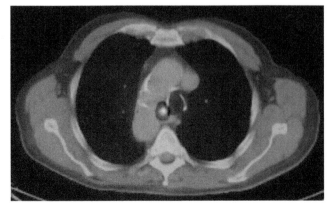

Fig. 8.9a *Cross-sectional PET-CT scan of the thorax showing an active station 4L lymph node.*

Fig. 8.9b *Cross-sectional PET-CT scan flipped left to right with the active station 4L lymph node.*

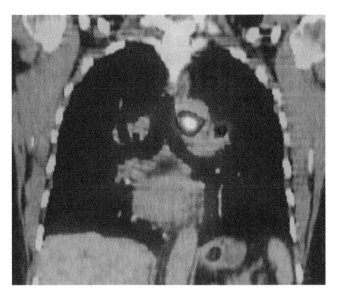

Fig. 8.9c *Coronal section of PET-CT scan showing the 4L lymph node.*

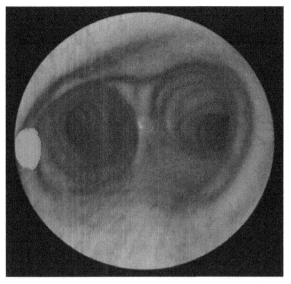

Fig. 8.9d *Bronchoscopic view of where the ultrasound probe should be placed to view the station 4L lymph nodes highlighted.*

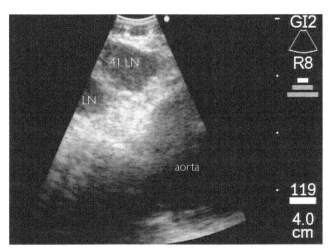

Fig. 8.9e *Ultrasound images of the station 4L lymph nodes.*

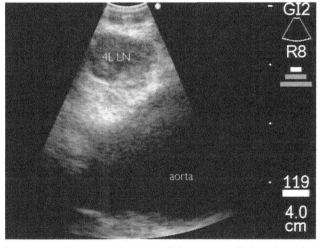

Fig. 8.9f *Ultrasound images of the station 4L lymph nodes with the aorta visible superior and distal to the nodes.*

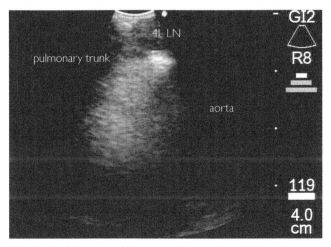

Fig. 8.9g *Ultrasound images of the station 4L lymph nodes with the aorta visible superior to, and the pulmonary trunk on the inferior aspect of, the nodes.*

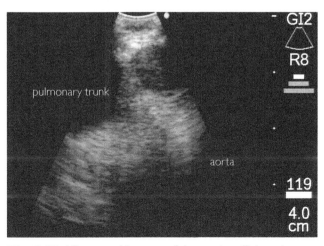

Fig. 8.9h *Ultrasound images of the station 4L lymph nodes with a greater portion of the pulmonary trunk visible.*

Station 5: Aortopulmonary lymph nodes (Fig. 8.10)

Station 5 can be visualized on endobronchial ultrasound but cannot routinely be sampled. The nodes are located between the aorta and the pulmonary artery lateral to the ligamentum arteriosum. On endobronchial ultrasound, the lymph node appears to be lying more peripheral to the pulmonary artery.

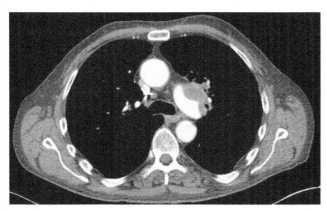

Fig. 8.10a *Cross-sectional CT scan of the thorax showing a station 5 lymph node.*

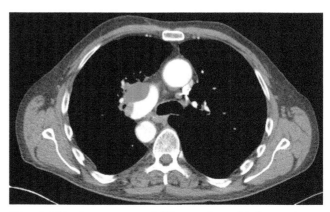

Fig. 8.10b *Cross-sectional CT scan flipped left to right with the active station 5 lymph node highlighted.*

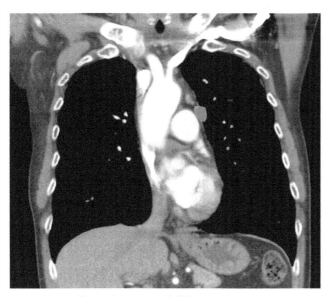

Fig. 8.10c *Coronal section of CT scan showing the station 5 lymph node highlighted.*

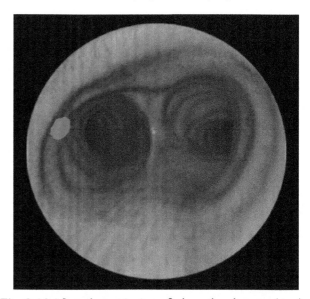

Fig. 8.10d *Bronchoscopic view of where the ultrasound probe should be placed to view the station 5 lymph nodes highlighted.*

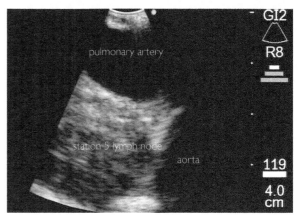

Fig. 8.10e *Ultrasound image of the station 5 lymph node visible distal to the pulmonary artery. The aorta is partly visible superiorly.*

Station 6: Para-aortic lymph nodes (Fig. 8.11)

The para-aortic lymph nodes, or station 6, may be visible on endobronchial ultrasound on the outer aspect of the ascending aorta and aortic arch, but again cannot be routinely sampled. The depth of ultrasound may need to be increased and, consequently, degradation of the image quality may make it difficult to visualize these lymph nodes.

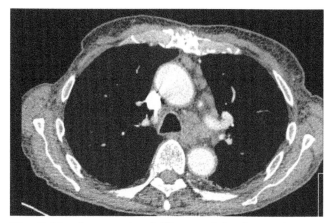

Fig. 8.11a *Cross-sectional CT scan of the thorax showing a station 6 lymph node.*

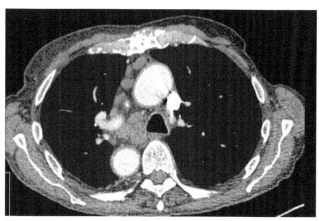

Fig. 8.11b *Cross-sectional CT scan flipped left to right with the active station 6 lymph node highlighted.*

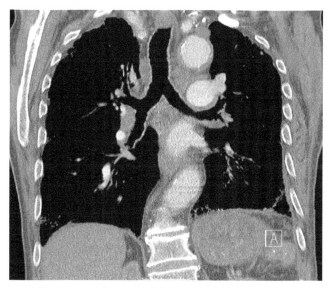

Fig. 8.11c *Coronal section of PET-CT scan showing the station 6 lymph node.*

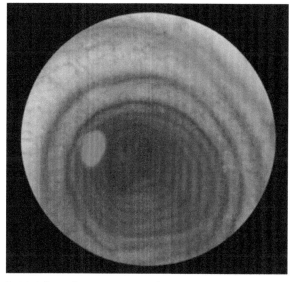

Fig. 8.11d *Bronchoscopic view of where the ultrasound probe should be placed to view the station 6 lymph nodes highlighted.*

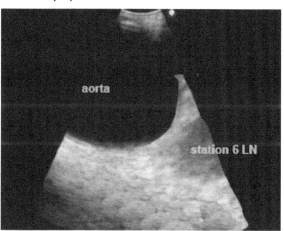

Fig. 8.11e *Ultrasound image of the station 6 lymph node.*

● Inferior mediastinal lymph nodes

Station 7: Subcarinal lymph node (Fig. 8.12)

The borders of station 7 are more clearly defined by the bronchoscopic view. It represents the nodal area inferior to the carina and down to the level where the right middle lobe bronchus originates on the right side and the secondary carina on the left side. The ultrasound transducer may be applied to the medial aspect of either the right or the left main bronchus. At this level, anterior movement of the transducer demonstrates the pulmonary artery and pulmonary trunk.

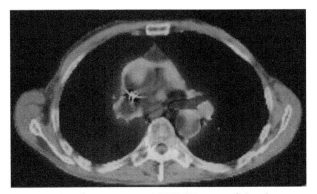

Fig. 8.12a *Cross-sectional PET-CT scan of the thorax showing a station 7 lymph node.*

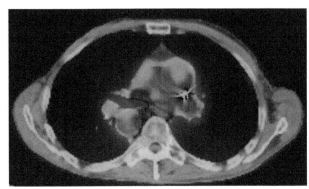

Fig. 8.12b *Cross-sectional PET-CT scan flipped left to right with the active station 7 lymph node.*

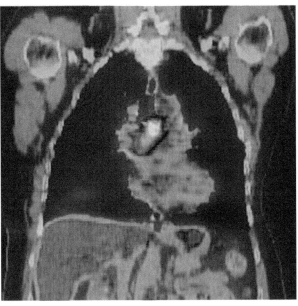

Fig. 8.12c *Coronal section of PET-CT scan showing the station 7 lymph node.*

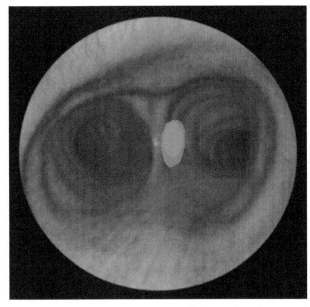

Fig. 8.12d *Bronchoscopic view of where the ultrasound probe should be placed to view the station 7 lymph nodes highlighted.*

Fig. 8.12e *Ultrasound image of the station 7 lymph node with its characteristic bean shape.*

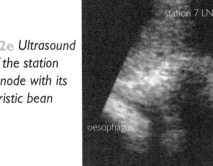

Fig. 8.12f *Ultrasound image of the station 7 lymph node with the oesophagus visible distally.*

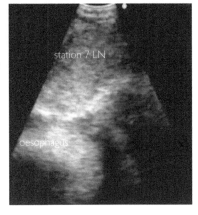

● Hilar zone lymph nodes

Station 10R: Right main bronchial lymph node (Fig. 8.13)

These lymph nodes are located at the right main bronchus. The upper border is defined by the position of the azygos vein, which should be identified on ultrasound, and the lower margin is the origin of the right upper lobe bronchus, which is identified on the broncho-scopic image. The transducer is applied on the anterior aspect of the right main bron-chus and slowly advanced. On ultrasound the structure that is visible on the anterior aspect includes the right pulmonary artery and, more peripheral to that, the superior vena cava.

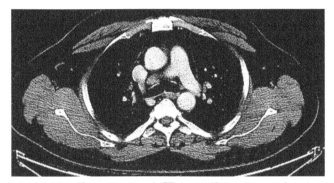

Fig. 8.13a *Cross-sectional CT scan of the thorax showing a station 10R lymph node.*

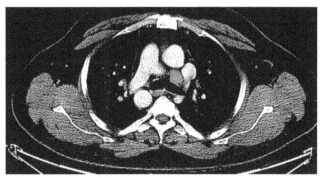

Fig. 8.13b *Cross-sectional CT scan flipped left to right with the station 10R lymph node highlighted.*

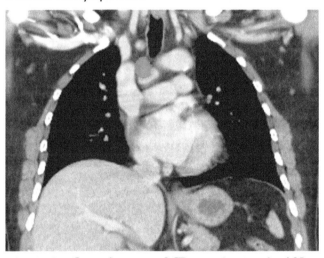

Fig. 8.13c *Coronal section of CT scan showing the 10R lymph node.*

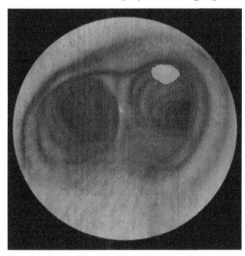

Fig. 8.13d *Bronchoscopic view of where the ultrasound probe should be placed to view the station 10R lymph nodes highlighted.*

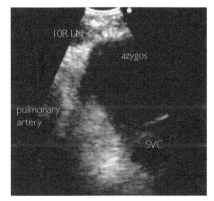

Fig. 8.13e *Ultrasound images of the station 10R lymph node: with the azygos visible, which delineates the border between station 4R and 10R.*

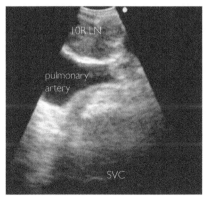

Fig. 8.13f *Ultrasound images of the station 10R lymph node: in a more central position.*

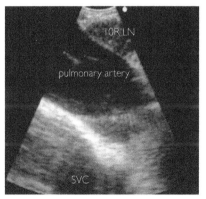

Fig. 8.13g *Ultrasound images of the station 10R lymph node: with the right pulmonary artery inferior and distal to the node.*

Station 10L: Left main bronchial lymph node (Fig. 8.14)

These are lymph nodes located on the left main bronchus. The upper border is again just below the carina on the left side and on ultrasound image is defined by the superior aspect of the pulmonary artery. The lower margin is indicated by the bifurcation of the left main bronchus into the superior lobar bronchus and the left lower lobe. The transducer should usually be applied to the anterior aspect of the left main bronchus and advanced slowly down towards the secondary carina. The structure visible anterior to the left main bronchus consists of the left pulmonary artery and trunk, and more inferiorly the left atrium may also be visible. On the medial aspect of the left main bronchus, the descending aorta may also be visible.

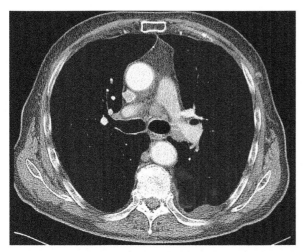

Fig. 8.14a *Cross-sectional CT scan of the thorax showing a station 10L lymph node.*

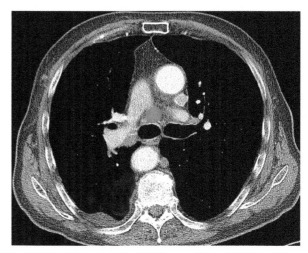

Fig. 8.14b *Cross-sectional CT scan flipped left to right with the station 10L lymph node highlighted.*

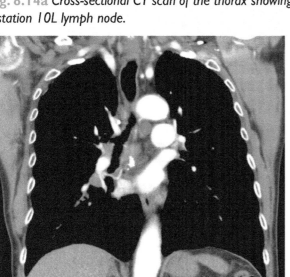

Fig. 8.14c *Coronal section of CT scan showing the 10L lymph node.*

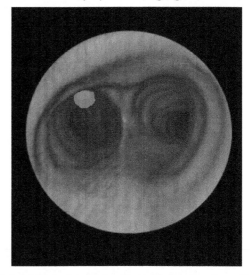

Fig. 8.14d *Bronchoscopic view with the location of station 10L lymph nodes highlighted.*

Fig. 8.14e *Ultrasound image of the station 10L lymph node with the pulmonary artery more superior and distal to the nodes. The pulmonary artery demarcates the 4L and 10L nodes.*

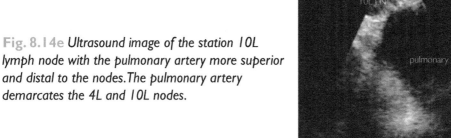

Station 11Rs: Right superior hilar lymph node (Fig. 8.15)

These are located at the upper lobe carina. The ultrasound transducer is applied just below the upper lobe origin in the bronchus intermedius. Superior to the 11R lymph node, the right upper lobe bronchus and pulmonary artery may be visible. Inferiorly the pulmonary artery branch and, more distally, the right pulmonary vein and superior vena cava are visible.

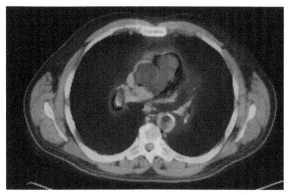

Fig. 8.15a *Cross-sectional PET-CT scan of the thorax showing a station 11Rs (right upper hilar) lymph node.*

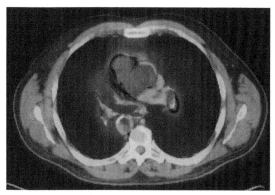

Fig. 8.15b *Cross-sectional PET-CT scan of the thorax flipped left to right showing the station 11Rs lymph node.*

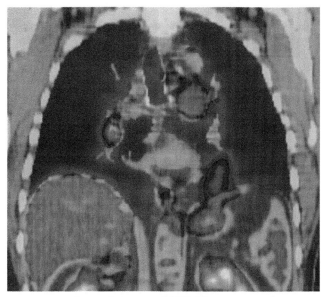

Fig. 8.15c *Coronal section of PET-CT scan showing the 11Rs lymph node.*

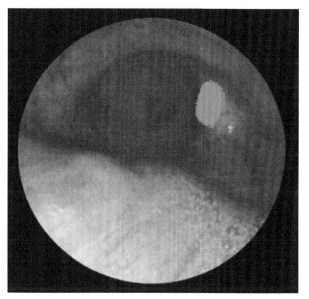

Fig. 8.15d *Bronchoscopic view of where the ultrasound probe should be placed to view the station 11Rs lymph nodes highlighted.*

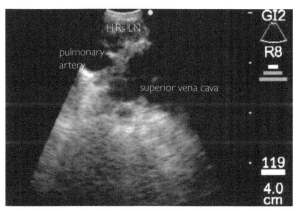

Fig. 8.15e *Ultrasound images of the station 11Rs lymph node: with the superior vena cava visible superior and distal to the nodes.*

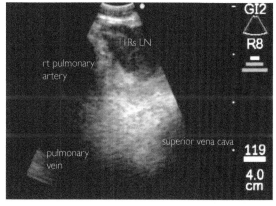

Fig. 8.15f *Ultrasound images of the station 11Rs lymph node: with the right pulmonary artery and vein visible inferior to the nodes.*

Station 11Ri: Right inferior hilar lymph node (Fig. 8.16)

These nodes are located at the distal aspect of the bronchus intermedius. They are lateral to the right middle lobe; anteriorly at this level the left atrium and right pulmonary vein are visible on the ultrasound images.

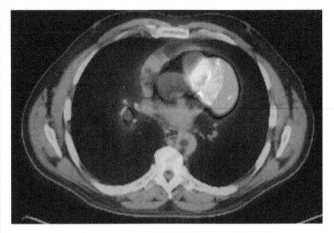

Fig. 8.16a *Cross-sectional PET-CT scan of the thorax showing a station 11Ri (right lower hilar) lymph node.*

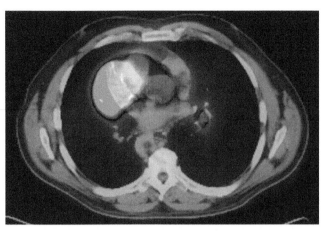

Fig. 8.16b *Cross-sectional PET-CT scan of the thorax flipped left to right showing the station 11Ri lymph node.*

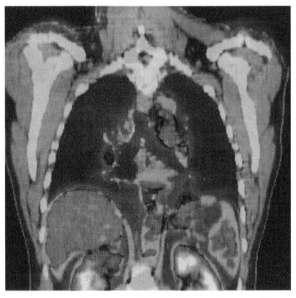

Fig. 8.16c *Coronal section of PET-CT scan showing the 11Ri lymph node.*

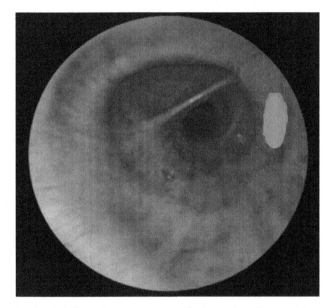

Fig. 8.16d *Bronchoscopic view of where the ultrasound probe should be placed to view the station 11Ri lymph nodes highlighted.*

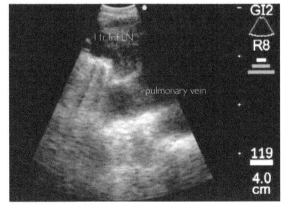

Fig. 8.16e *Ultrasound image of the station 11Ri lymph node.*

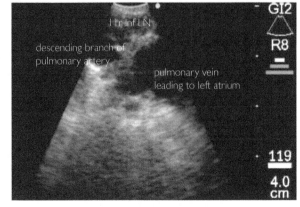

Fig. 8.16f *Station 11Ri lymph node with the pulmonary vein which leads to the left atrium.*

Station 11L: Left hilar lymph node (Fig. 8.17)

These nodes are at the secondary carina on the left side between the left lower lobe and the left upper lobe bronchus. The left pulmonary artery and left pulmonary veins are usually visible anteriorly in this location.

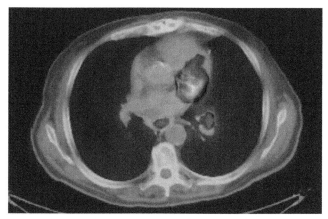

Fig. 8.17a *Cross-sectional PET-CT scan of the thorax showing a station 11L lymph node.*

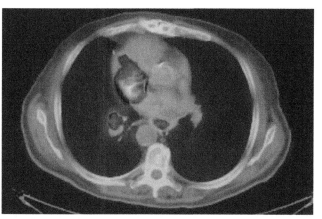

Fig. 8.17b *Cross-sectional PET-CT scan of the thorax flipped left to right showing a station 11L lymph node.*

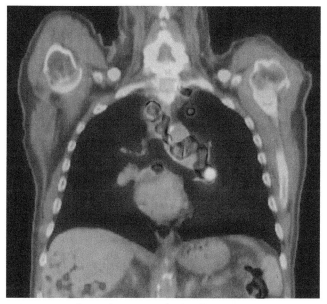

Fig. 8.17c *Coronal section of PET-CT scan showing the 11L lymph node.*

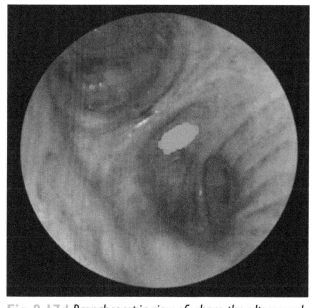

Fig. 8.17d *Bronchoscopic view of where the ultrasound probe should be placed to view the station 11L lymph nodes highlighted.*

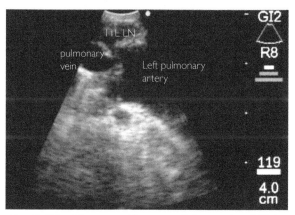

Fig. 8.17e *Ultrasound images of the station 11L lymph node: with left pulmonary artery and left upper lobe bronchus more superior.*

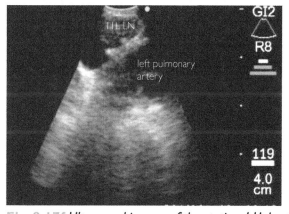

Fig. 8.17f *Ultrasound images of the station 11L lymph node: with the lingular bronchus visible inferior to the node.*

Lymph node sampling

As in conventional TBNA, the highest lymph node stations should be sampled, i.e. any contralateral hilar or mediastinal lymph nodes (N3 station lymph nodes) followed by N2 lymph nodes and finally any hilar lymph nodes. Any paratracheal tumour masses can also be sampled but should be sampled only after any visible N3 or N2 lymph nodes have been sampled. This minimizes the risk of false-positive results to almost zero and prevents falsely upstaging a patient with lung cancer. Only the recommended needles should be used with ultrasound bronchoscope – they are specially designed for the bronchoscope and the use of alternative needles may lead to puncture of the working channel of this very expensive instrument.

● *Technique*

The needle length and position can be set prior to insertion of the bronchoscope into the patient. However, we recommend verifying that the needle sheath is visible outside the instrument channel bronchoscope each time the needle is inserted through the working channel of the bronchoscope and prior to any needle aspiration. The needle should be fixed in position so that a small crescent of the sheath is visible on the endotracheal image (Fig. 8.18). This will minimize instrument channel damage and significantly prolong the life and service of your ultrasound bronchoscope.

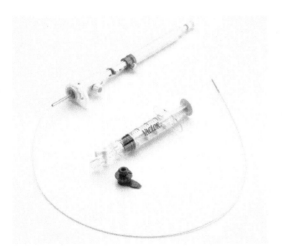

Fig. 8.18a *Specific needle for the Olympus endobronchial bronchoscope.*

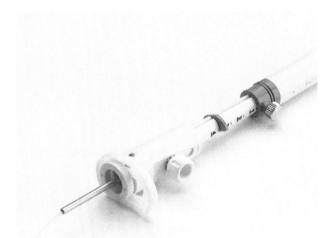

Fig. 8.18b *Close-up of the handle of the needle showing the mechanism for the adjustment of the needle sheath.*

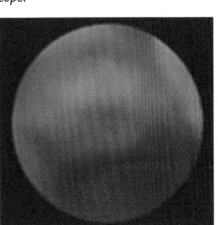

Fig. 8.18c *Bronchoscopic image showing the small crescent of the sheath which should be visible prior to attempted needle aspiration. This shows the ideal position.*

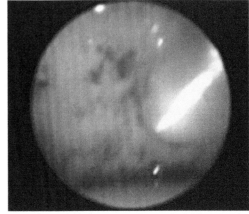

Fig. 8.18d *Bronchoscopic image showing the significant length of the visible sheath. This greater distance may impair acoustic contact and hence the ultrasound image.*

The needle should be introduced into the bronchoscope straight into the trachea. The needle tip should be adjusted so that a very small crescent is visible in the endoscopic image on the top right-hand corner. Once the lymph node or mass is identified in the ultrasound field, an assistant is asked to secure the bronchoscope and hold it in position. The central stylet is then withdrawn about 3 mm so that the needle point is sharp. The safety lock for the needle is lowered to the required distance and the needle gently inserted through the airway wall whilst maintaining the ultrasound image at all times (Figs 8.19 and 8.20). Once the needle is through the airway wall into the lymph node, the stylet is jiggled back and forth in order to remove any cartilage or airway wall plug from the needle. The stylet is then removed and the aspiration syringe connected. The syringe is preset with suction and, providing it is within the lymph node, the three-way tap is opened and the needle moved gently back and forth through the lymph node. This allows cellular material from the lymph node to be aspirated. The bronchoscope can be gently manipulated so that material from different parts of the lymph node is aspirated. The three-way tap is then closed and the needle withdrawn back into the sheath and the needle removed.

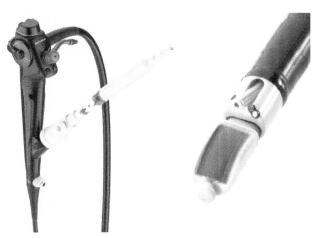

Fig. 8.19a *Endobronchial ultrasound bronchoscope with the needle fixed in position on the scope.*

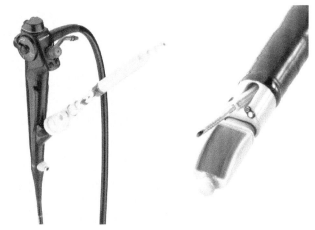

Fig. 8.19b *Endobronchial ultrasound bronchoscope with the needle protruding out at the distal tip of the bronchoscope.*

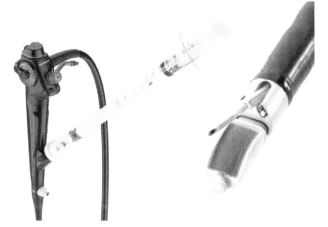

Fig. 8.19c *Endobronchial ultrasound bronchoscope with the needle protruding out, syringe attached distally and suction on. The needle is then gently pushed back and forth in the lymph node.*

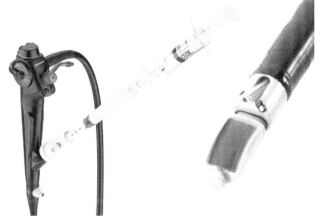

Fig. 8.19d *Endobronchial ultrasound bronchoscope with the suction off on the attached syringe and the needle withdrawn back.*

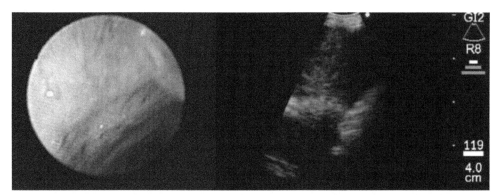

Fig. 8.20a *Bronchoscopic view of the needle sheath and ultrasound image of the lymph node.*

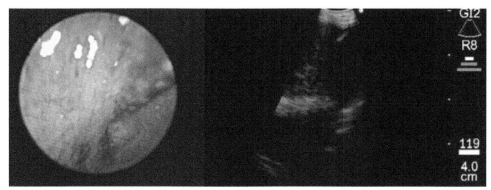

Fig. 8.20b *Bronchoscopic view of the needle tip and ultrasound image of the lymph node showing initial penetration of the needle.*

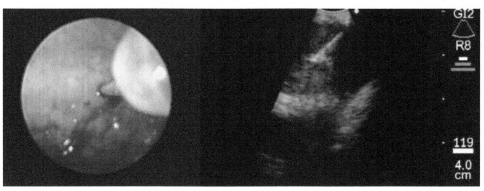

Fig. 8.20c *Bronchoscopic view of the needle tip and sheath with the corresponding ultrasound image of the lymph node showing needle aspiration of the lymph node.*

The material that has been aspirated in the needle can be either smeared on to slides or fixed or injected into saline for liquid cytology media (Fig. 8.21). You should discuss the preparation with your pathologists so that samples that are suited to the local practice are collected. Placing the cellular material in saline or liquid cytology media allows more professional slides to be prepared and furthermore allows the material to be spun down into a cell pellet which can be further evaluated by histology. Immunohistochemistry can also be performed on the cell blocks to optimally classify any malignant cells identified and also characterize the genotype in the biopsy material.

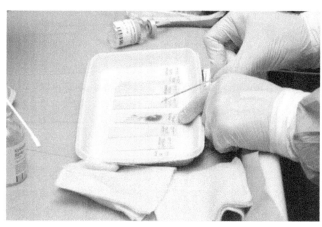

Fig. 8.21a *Lymph node aspirate is injected on to a glass slide.*

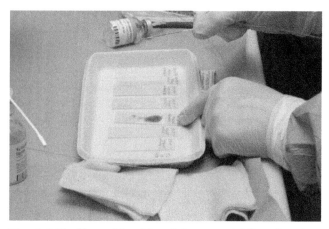

Fig. 8.21b *Glass slide with cellular material from lymph node aspiration.*

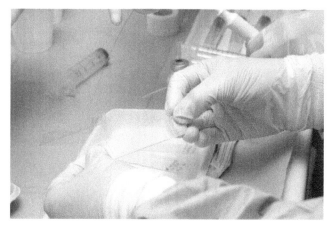

Fig. 8.21c *The glass slide with cellular material is gently apposed to another glass slide and then slid apart to create a thin smear on the slide.*

CHAPTER 9

Pathology

This chapter consists mainly of bronchoscopic images of the various pathological conditions encountered during bronchoscopy. The sections cover pathology seen on the vocal cords through to the trachea, lobar bronchi and bronchial segments.

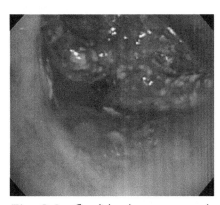

Fig. 9.1a *Candida plaques on vocal cords in a patient on inhaled steroids.*

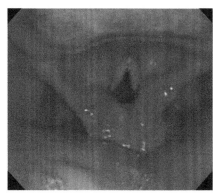

Fig. 9.1b *Paralysed left vocal cord. Note the left vocal cord is in the midline position.*

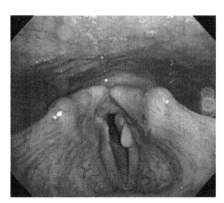

Fig. 9.1c *Vocal cord polyp.*

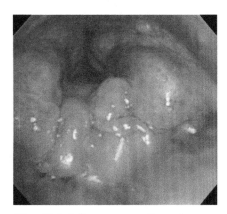

Fig. 9.1d *Squamous cell carcinoma involving the vocal cords.*

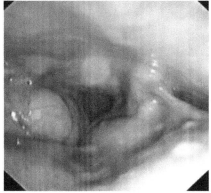

Fig. 9.1e *Vocal cords infiltrated by amyloid (primary tracheobronchial amyloid, AL type).*

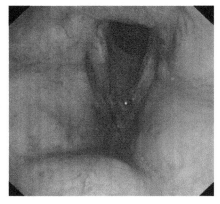

Fig. 9.1f *Limited Kaposi's sarcoma involving vocal cord.*

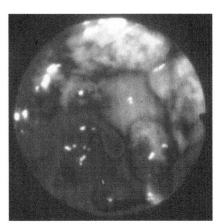

Fig. 9.1g *Severe Kaposi's sarcoma involving vocal cord.*

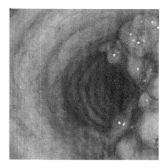

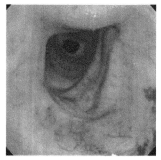

Fig. 9.2a *Distorted trachea with deviation of the upper trachea towards the right with the tracheal web in the distal aspect.*

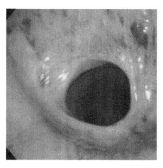

Fig. 9.2b *Tracheal web.*

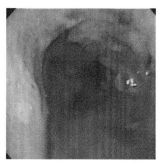

Fig. 9.2c *Adenocarcinoma of the trachea.*

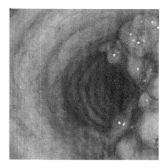

Fig. 9.2d *Adenocystic carcinoma involving the trachea.*

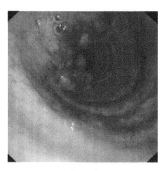

Fig. 9.2e *Poorly differentiated carcinoma infiltrating through the mid-trachea.*

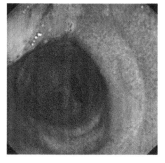

Fig. 9.2f *Tracheo-oesophageal fistula in a patient with oesophageal carcinoma undergoing radiotherapy.*

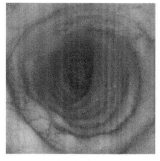

Fig. 9.2g *Some cartilage nodules on the trachea in the anterior aspect.*

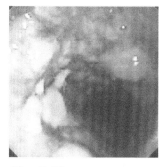

Fig. 9.2h *Tracheobronchopathia osteochondroplastica: acute inflammatory stage.*

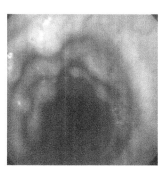

Fig. 9.2i *Tracheobronchopathia osteochondroplastica: chronic stage with thickening of the cartilaginous portions of the trachea.*

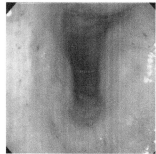

Fig. 9.2j *Sabre trachea.*

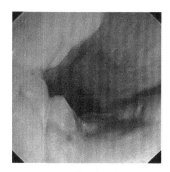

Fig. 9.2k *Tracheobronchial amyloid with greater involvement of the anterior aspect of the trachea.*

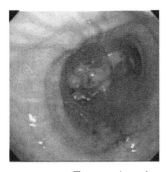

Fig. 9.3a *Tumour (renal cell carcinoma) involving the carina and almost completely occluding both main bronchi.*

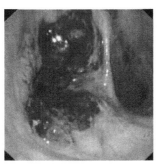

Fig. 9.3b *Extrinsic tumour circumferential involving the right main bronchus at the level of the carina.*

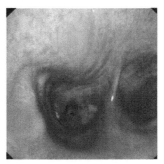

Fig. 9.3c *Widening of the carina due to tumour involving the subcarinal lymph node. Note the infiltration of the mucosa in the medial aspect of the right main bronchus.*

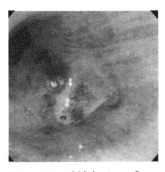

Fig. 9.3d *Widening of the carina and complete occlusion of the left main bronchus by tumour.*

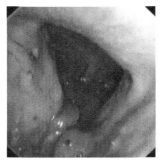

Fig. 9.3e *Tracheobronchial amyloid involving the carina. Note the thickened nodular plaque-like aggregations.*

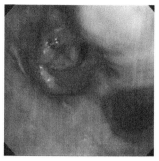

Fig. 9.4a *Polypoid non-small-cell carcinoma originating from the right upper lobe and occluding the right main bronchus.*

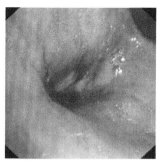

Fig. 9.4b *Invasive squamous cell carcinoma originating from the posterior wall of the right main bronchus.*

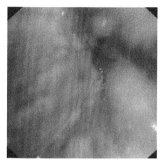

Fig. 9.4c *Circumferential tumour (adenocarcinoma) occluding the right lower lobe bronchus.*

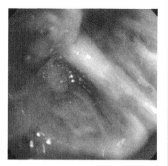

Fig. 9.4d *Segmental tumour (adenocarcinoma) occluding the anterior segment (RB3) of the right upper lobe.*

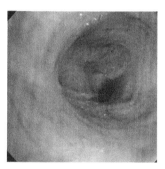

Fig. 9.4e *Concentric segmental tumour (adenocarcinoma) involving the lateral segment of the left lower lobe (LB9).*

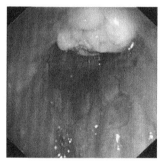

Fig. 9.4f *Polypoid non-small cell carcinoma originating from the apical segment of the right upper lobe (RB1).*

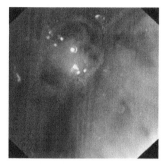

Fig. 9.4g *Small cell carcinoma occluding the right upper lobe.*

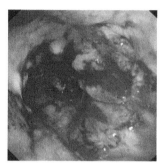

Fig. 9.4h *Diffuse infiltrative carcinoma involving the left main bronchus.*

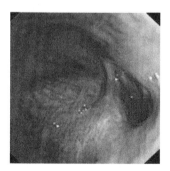

Fig. 9.4i *Extrinsic compression of the right upper lobe from extrabronchial tumour.*

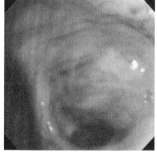

Fig. 9.4j *Extrinsic tumour bulging and partly occluding the apical segment of the right upper lobe (RB6).*

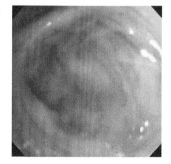

Fig. 9.4k *Complete occlusion of the apical segment of the left lower lobe (LB6) from an extrinsic tumour.*

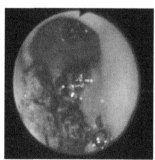

Fig. 9.4l *Kaposi's sarcoma involving secondary carina of the left lower lobe (LC2).*

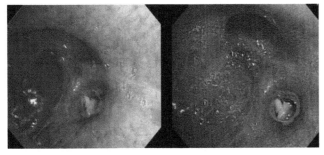

Fig. 9.5a *Polypoid necrotic tumour originating from the posterior segment of the right upper lobe (RB2) and extrinsic compression of the anterior segment of the right upper lobe (RB3). Left: video bronchoscopy image; right: narrow-band imaging. Increased vascularity is evident in the extrinsic lesion and lack of blood vessels in the necrotic tumour.*

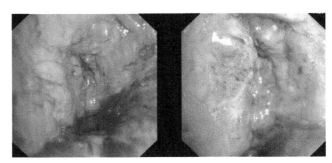

Fig. 9.5b *Small cell carcinoma involving the right upper lobe with increased tortuosity of blood vessels and blind-ending punctate vessels.*

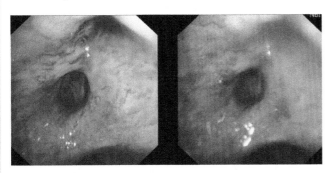

Fig. 9.5c *Squamous cell carcinoma involving the apical segment of the left lower lobe following treatment with radiotherapy. Note the increased inflammatory changes and increased capillary loops.*

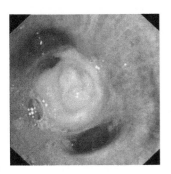

Fig. 9.6a *Metastatic colorectal carcinoma involving the right basal bronchus.*

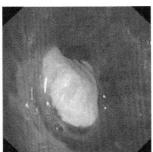

Fig. 9.6b *Metastatic colonic carcinoma occluding the left main bronchus.*

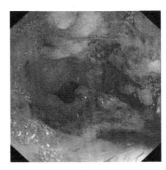

Fig. 9.6c *Infiltrating oesophageal adenocarcinoma involving the right main bronchus.*

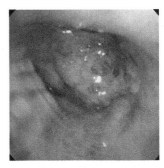

Fig. 9.6d *Metastatic endometrial carcinoma involving the left lower lobe.*

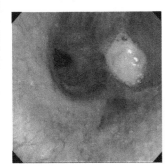

Fig. 9.6e *Renal cell carcinoma involving the left main bronchus.*

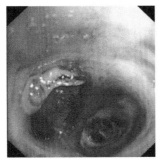

Fig. 9.6f *Hurthle cell carcinoma involving the segmental bronchus in the right middle lobe.*

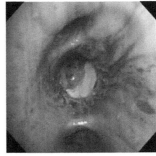

Fig. 9.6g *Leiomyosarcoma involving the lateral segment of the left lower lobe (LB9).*

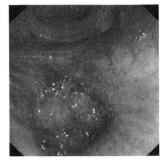

Fig. 9.6h *Squamous cell carcinoma from a metastatic head and neck carcinoma involving the left main bronchus.*

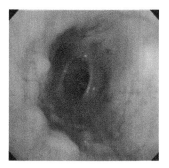

Fig. 9.7a *Nodules giving a cobblestone appearance in the right lower lobe from sarcoid.*

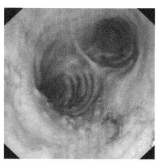

Fig. 9.7b *Nodularity around the lower trachea due to tuberculosis.*

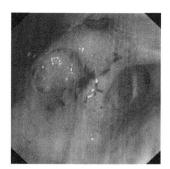

Fig. 9.7c *Tuberculous granuloma occluding the anterior segment of the right upper lobe (RB3).*

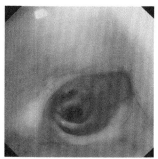

Fig. 9.7d *Anthracosis (darkened) area in the medial aspect, which is occasionally seen in patients with pulmonary tuberculosis.*

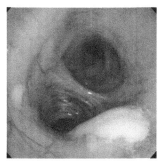

Fig. 9.7e *Mucus originating from the segmental bronchus.*

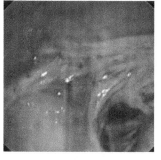

Fig. 9.7f *Mucus plugging due to allergic bronchopulmonary aspergillosis.*

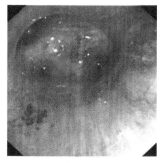

Fig. 9.7g *Concentric narrowing of upper lobe segments in a patient with allergic bronchopulmonary aspergillosis.*

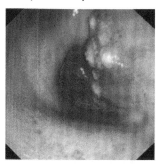

Fig. 9.7h *Pith-like lesions in the bronchus intermedius due to bronchocentric granulomatosis.*

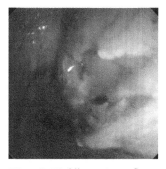

Fig. 9.7i *Ulceration of pith-filled lesions after steroid treatment in a patient with bronchocentric granulomatosis.*

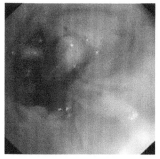

Fig. 9.7j *Granulation tissue which has developed secondary to a foreign body.*

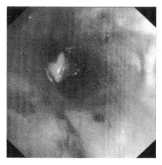

Fig. 9.7k *Foreign body (tooth) in the right main bronchus.*

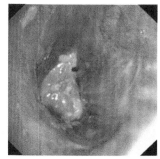

Fig. 9.7l *A tooth visible in the right lower lobe of a patient presenting with recurrent lobar pneumonia.*

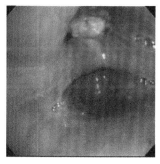

Fig. 9.7m *Inflammatory pseudo-tumour.*

163

Fluorescence-based imaging

Autofluorescence bronchoscopy

All epithelial tissue has an innate fluorescence but this is not discernible without some enhancement. With autofluorescence bronchoscopy the airways are illuminated with a blue light (395–445 nm). The autofluorescence signal (550 nm) is incorporated in the video processor with the other reflected light to form a composite image where normal tissue appears as green (fluorescent tissue). Any reduction in fluorescence shows up as a pink through to magenta colour. Blood appears dark green (Fig. 10.1). Care should be taken as any mucus or secretions overlying the epithelial tissue conceal the normal fluorescent epithelium and falsely appear pink. Autofluorescence bronchoscopy requires a special bronchoscope and usually the mode can be switched from white light to fluorescence by simply pressing a remote button on the bronchoscope or a foot pedal.

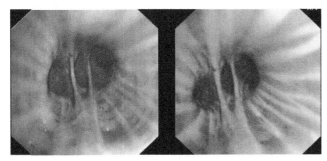

Fig. 10.1a *Video bronchoscopy and fluorescence bronchoscopy image of the left lower lobe.*

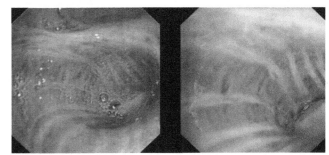

Fig. 10.1b *Mucus secretions in the right middle lobe which appear pink and can be easily mistaken for an abnormal area.*

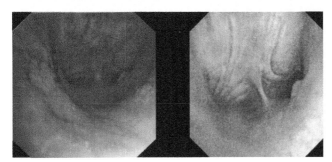

Fig. 10.1c *Loss of fluorescence in the inflammatory nodule in the lower trachea.*

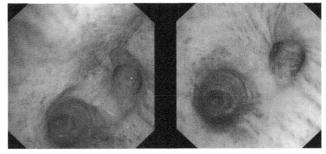

Fig. 10.1d *Abnormal fluorescence of the left main carina showing subtle abnormality not visible on video bronchoscopy.*

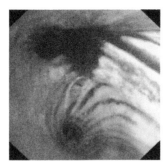

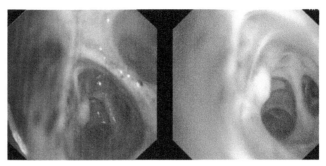

Fig. 10.1e *Blood appears dark green on fluorescence bronchoscopy.*

Fig. 10.1f *Cartilage nodule in the right lower lobe segment with normal fluorescence.*

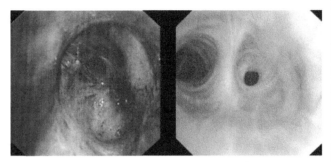

Fig. 10.1g *Inflammatory web with normal fluorescence in the left lower lobe.*

Fluorescence bronchoscopy is used primarily as a research tool. In some cases, where a patient has had multiple cancers (head and neck or lung cancer) or where there are multiple areas of field effect (patchy change in airways from metaplasia through to carcinoma in situ), the patients undergo regular fluorescence bronchoscopy for clinical surveillance. These patients may undergo repeated bronchoscopy over several years and possibly by several operators. Hence, careful documentation is essential and standard nomenclature is required to describe the location and extent of the abnormalities (Fig. 10.2). We would recommend use of nomenclature as in Chapter 2.

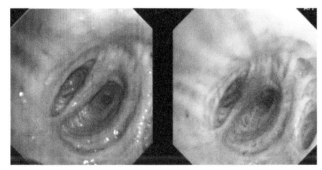

Fig. 10.2a *Thickening of the carina with abnormal fluorescence between the lateral segment of the left lower lobe (LB9) and the posterior segment of the left lower lobe (LB10) due to mild dysplasia.*

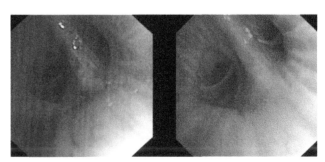

Fig. 10.2b *Thickening of the carina with abnormal fluorescence between the anterior segment of the right lower lobe (RB8) and the lateral segment of the right lower lobe (RB9) due to moderate dysplasia.*

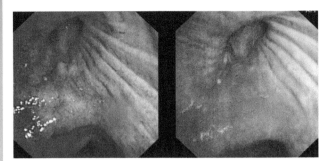

Fig. 10.2c *Nodularity with abnormal fluorescence in the inferior aspect of the right upper lobe carina due to severe dysplasia.*

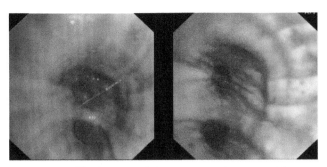

Fig. 10.2d *Thickening of the segmental carina with abnormal fluorescence in the right lower lobe due to carcinoma in situ.*

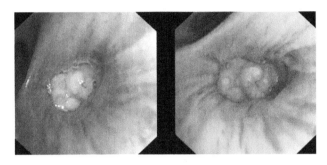

Fig. 10.2e *Abnormal fluorescence of polypoid tumour in the apical segment of the left lower lobe.*

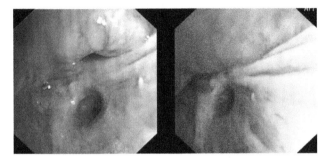

Fig. 10.2f *Tumour around the apical segment of the right upper lobe and some narrowing of the anterior segment of the right upper lobe.*

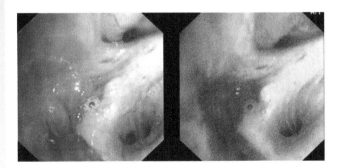

Fig. 10.2g *Tumour with abnormal fluorescence around the anterior segment of the right upper lobe.*

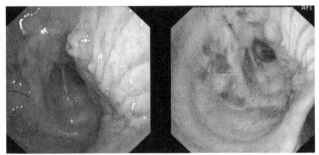

Fig. 10.2h *Right lower lobe sleeve resection with nodularity which appears suspicious on white light but has normal fluorescence. Patchy abnormal fluorescence due to secretions.*

Confocal microscopy

Confocal endomicroscopy is a fluorescence-based imaging technique which illuminates the airways or lung parenchyma with a blue argon laser light at a wavelength of 488 nm. The probe, which consists of a bundle of optical fibres, is inserted through the instrument channel of the bronchoscope (Fig. 10.3). The probe can be applied to the proximal airways for evaluating the trachea, main bronchi and bronchial segments (Fig. 10.4). The elastin, which is found in the basement membrane, provides information on the bronchial tree. The probe can be easily passed into a subsegment and slowly advanced from the lobular bronchus to the terminal bronchiole, the respiratory bronchiole and then to the alveolar acinus. Elastin is a structural connective tissue component of the alveolar walls and the confocal probe detects the fluorescent elastin scaffold of the lobule used to image the proximal airways and down to the alveoli.

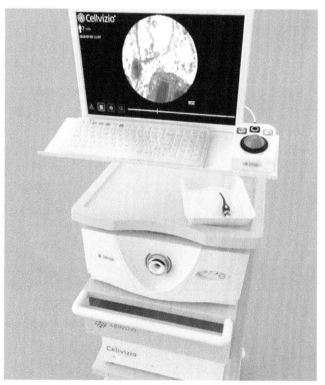

Fig. 10.3a *Cellvizio confocal microscopy system.*

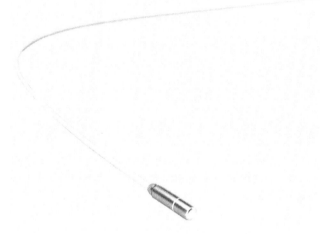

Fig. 10.3b *Confocal probe.*

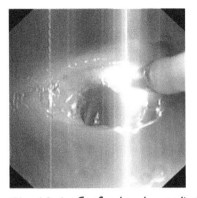

Fig. 10.4a *Confocal probe applied on the airway segment.*

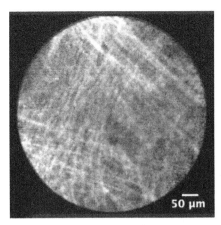

Fig. 10.4b *Confocal microscopy images of the bronchial segments showing the lattice network of elastin in the basement membrane.*

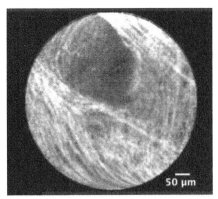

Fig. 10.4c *Confocal microscopy of a bronchial segment with an area without fluorescence due to a bronchial gland.*

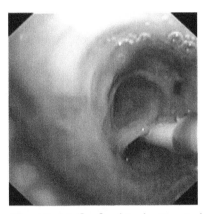

Fig. 10.4d *Confocal probe inserted into the bronchial segment and into lung parenchyma.*

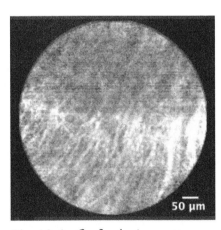

Fig. 10.4e *Confocal microscopy image of a bronchiole.*

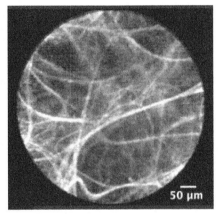

Fig. 10.4f *Normal alveoli with elastin scaffolding visible with confocal microscopy.*

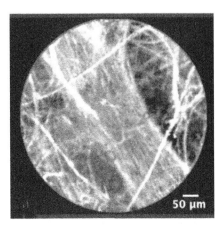

Fig. 10.4g *Normal blood vessel in alveoli.*

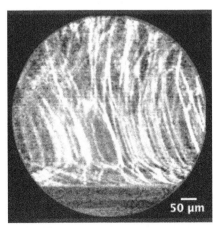

Fig. 10.4h *Normal pleura with longitudinal elastin network and fewer cross-linking fibres.*

Light radiating back from the fluorescing tissue between 500 and 650 nm is collected at 12 frames/second. This creates a high-quality real-time image with a diameter field of view of 600 μm but a depth of penetration of approximately 50 μm and a lateral resolution of 3.5 μm. This is a developing field and the images shown in Figs 10.5–10.8 are from the early research.

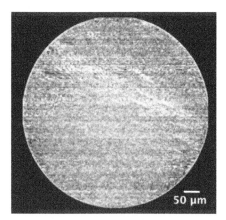

Fig. 10.5a *Loss of fluorescence and reticular pattern due to a bronchial tumour (squamous cell carcinoma).*

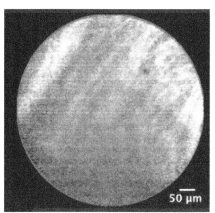

Fig. 10.5b *Edge of endobronchial tumour with some distortion of fluorescence pattern in the upper aspect and loss of fluorescence in the inferior aspect.*

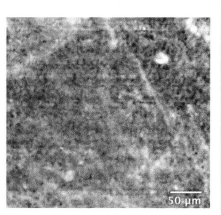

Fig. 10.5c *Loss of fluorescence from the alveolar architecture in bronchioloalveolar cell carcinoma.*

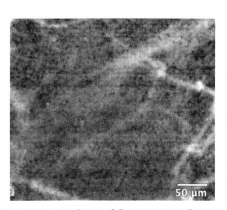

Fig. 10.5d *Loss of fluorescence from the alveolar architecture due to non-small cell lung cancer.*

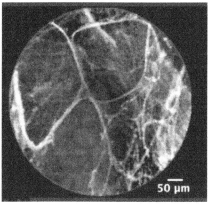

Fig. 10.6a *Confocal microscopy in a patient with moderate emphysema. Note the large cystic spaces.*

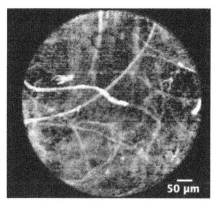

Fig. 10.6b *Disruption of elastin alveolar structure with large cystic areas in emphysema.*

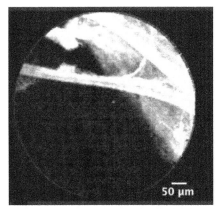

Fig. 10.6c *Large bulla in a patient with severe emphysema with some remaining alveolar structure in the superior aspect.*

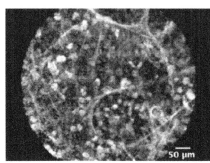

Fig. 10.6d *Fluorescent macrophages in the alveoli in a smoker with chronic obstructive pulmonary disease.*

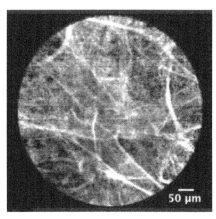

Fig. 10.7a *Thickened interstitium and increased elastin network in interstitial pneumonitis (pulmonary fibrosis).*

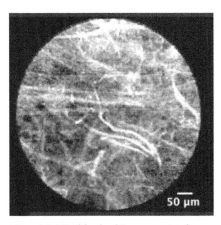

Fig. 10.7b *Marked increase in the elastin network with thickening of the alveoli in interstitial pneumonitis (pulmonary fibrosis).*

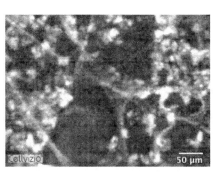

Fig. 10.7c *Increased fluorescent cells and some thickening of the elastin network in pulmonary sarcoidosis.*

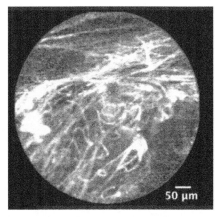

Fig. 10.7d *Abnormal spiral loops of elastin in a granuloma in a patient with sarcoidosis.*

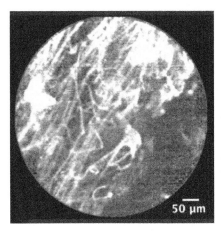

Fig. 10.7e *Further example of abnormal spiral loops of elastin in a granuloma due to sarcoidosis.*

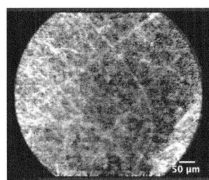

Fig. 10.7f *Increased fluorescent cells within normal elastin alveolar architecture in drug-related hypersensitivity pneumonitis.*

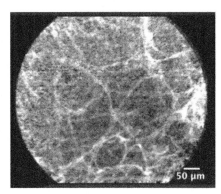

Fig. 10.7g *Drug-related hypersensitivity pneumonitis with normal elastin alveolar architecture and increased cellularity.*

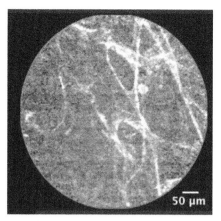

Fig. 10.8a *Reduced fluorescence of alveolar architecture due to consolidation from pneumonia.*

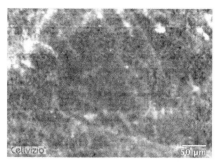

Fig. 10.8b *Alveolar architecture obscured by cells with low fluorescence in pneumonia.*

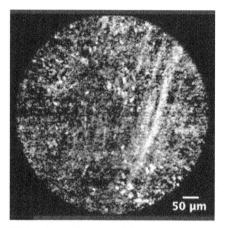

Fig. 10.8c *Increased fluorescent cells in organizing pneumonia.*

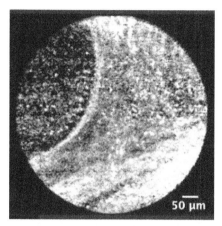

Fig. 10.8d *Increased fluorescent cells adjacent to a blood vessel in organizing pneumonia.*

Electromagnetic navigation

The superDimension® system (iLogic) is a real-time navigation system using an electromagnetic field to aid navigation to a particular target area (Fig. 11.1; the indications for its use are given in Box 11.1).

BOX 11.1 Indications for superDimension® navigation

- Sampling of peripheral nodule
- Guidance for transbronchial fine-needle aspiration of mediastinal lymph nodes and peribronchial masses
- Targeted transbronchial cryobiopsy
- Insertion of fiducial markers for stereotactic radiotherapy or cyberknife
- Insertion of markers for video-assisted thoracic surgical (VATS) biopsy

---

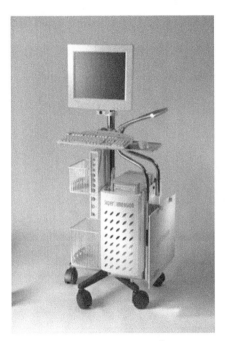

Fig. 11.1 *SuperDimension® system.*

Planning stage

The initial planning stage requires a multi-slice CT scan (2 mm with at least 1 mm overlap). The CT is then uploaded onto a planning module. A virtual bronchoscopy is performed on the planning module and important landmarks such as the main carina, right upper lobe carina, right middle lobe carina, left main carina and carina between the left basal segments and the apical segment of the left lower lobe (LC, LB6–LB8) are marked (Fig. 11.2).

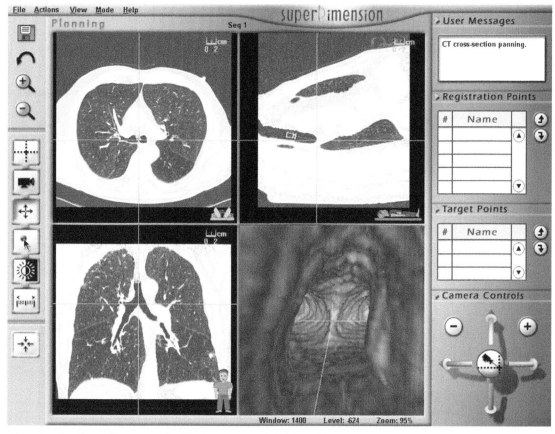

Fig. 11.2a *SuperDimension® CT planning module. Virtual bronchoscopy mode showing: carina.*

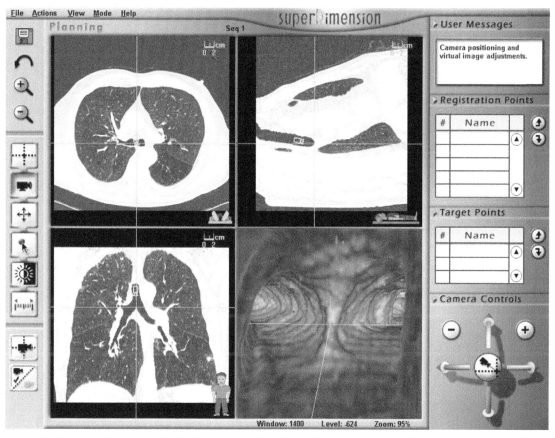

Fig. 11.2b *SuperDimension® CT planning module. Virtual bronchoscopy mode showing: close-up of carina.*

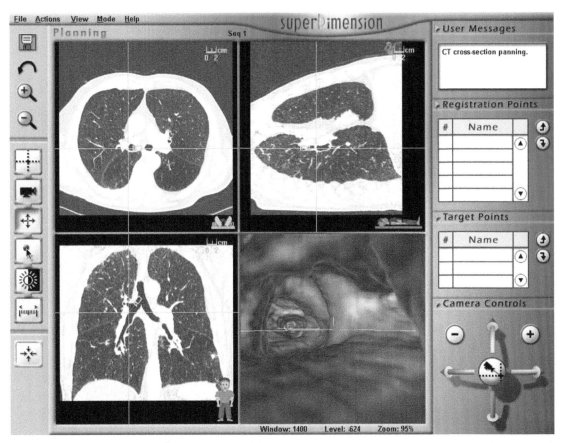

Fig. 11.2c *SuperDimension® CT planning module. Virtual bronchoscopy mode showing: right upper lobe. (RC1)*

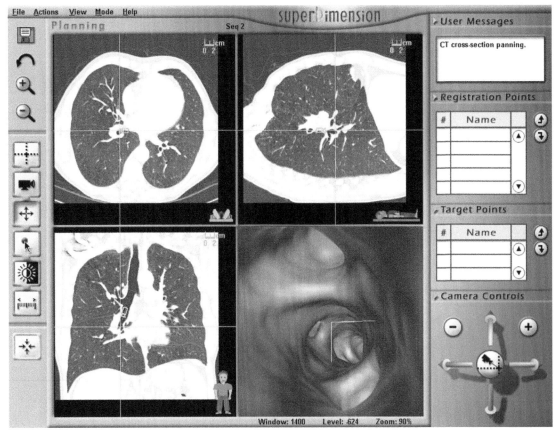

Fig. 11.2d *SuperDimension® CT planning module. Virtual bronchoscopy mode showing: right middle lobe (RC2).*

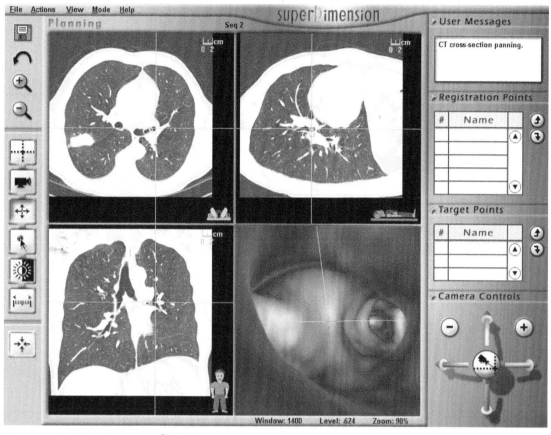

Fig. 11.2e *SuperDimension® CT planning module. Virtual bronchoscopy mode showing: left main carina (LC2).*

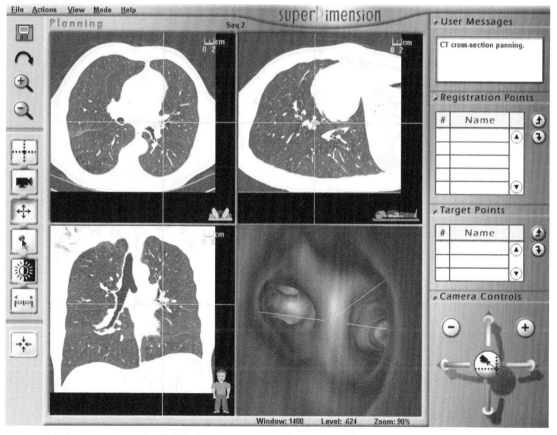

Fig. 11.2f *SuperDimension® CT planning module. Virtual bronchoscopy mode showing: carina of the left apical basal segment (LC LB6–LB8).*

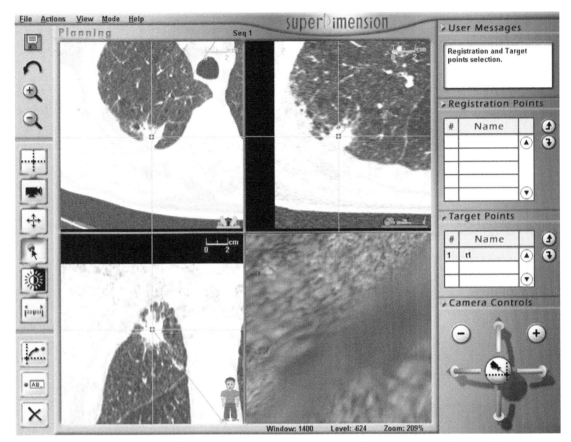

Fig. 11.2g *SuperDimension® CT planning module. Virtual bronchoscopy mode showing: the target located.*

The target areas are also marked on the planning module in the CT mode with or without intermediate markers (Fig. 11.3). The information for the planning module is exported and loaded onto the superDimension navigation module.

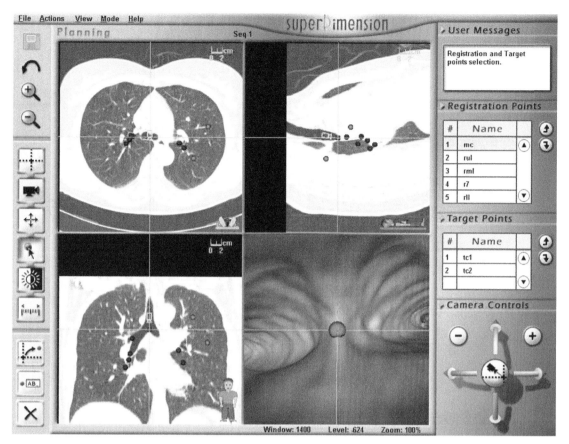

Fig. 11.3a *Marking of landmarks during virtual bronchoscopy on the superDimension® CT planning module: main carina.*

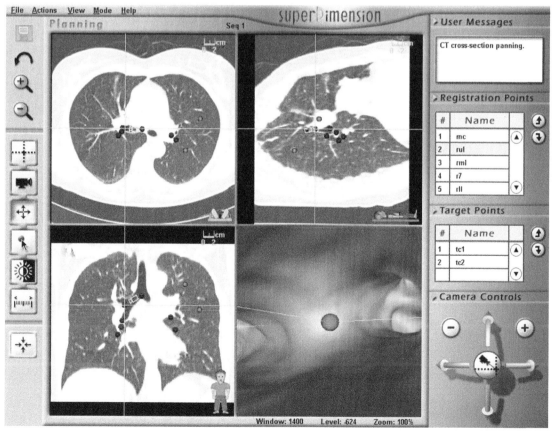

Fig. 11.3b *Marking of landmarks during virtual bronchoscopy on the superDimension® CT planning module: right upper lobe carina (RC1).*

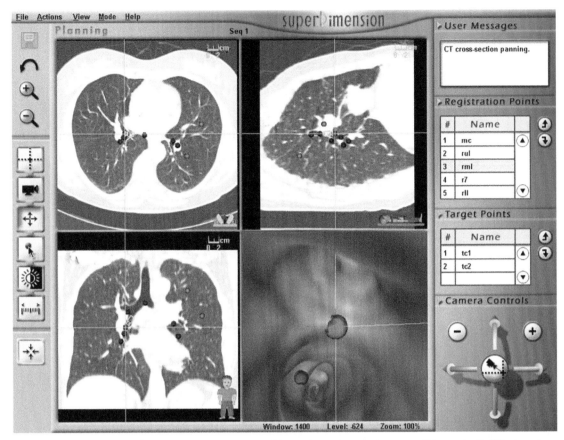

Fig. 11.3c *Marking of landmarks during virtual bronchoscopy on the superDimension® CT planning module: right middle lobe carina (RC2).*

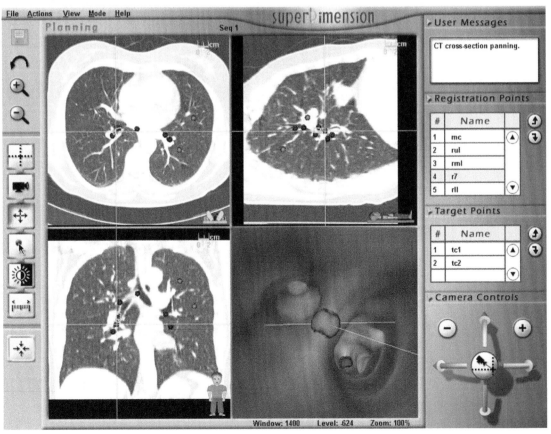

Fig. 11.3d *Marking of landmarks during virtual bronchoscopy on the superDimension® CT planning module: carina of the right apical basal segment marked (RC RB6–RB8).*

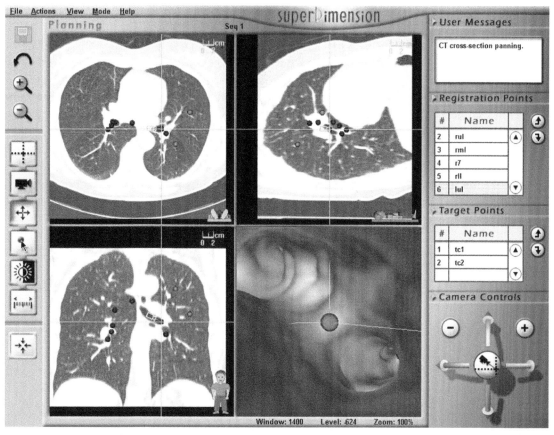

Fig. 11.3e *Marking of landmarks during virtual bronchoscopy on the superDimension® CT planning module: left secondary carina (LC2).*

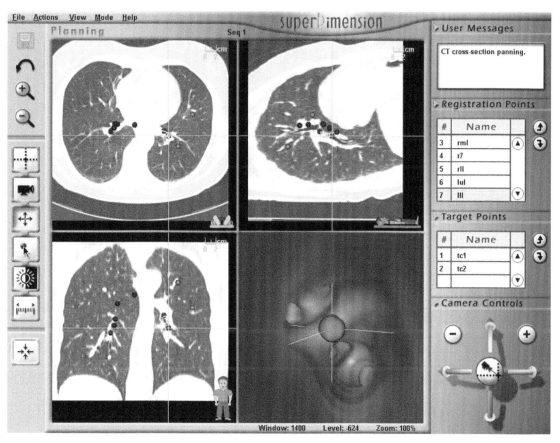

Fig. 11.3f *Marking of landmarks during virtual bronchoscopy on the superDimension® CT planning module: carina between the left apical basal (LB6) and basal segments (LC LB6–LB8).*

Registration process

The bronchoscopy is performed with the patient lying flat on an electromagnetic board (Fig. 11.4). This creates a magnetic field, and the electromagnetic tracker placed through the instrument channel of the bronchoscope can be used to detect the position of the tip in this electromagnetic field. The navigation phase involves registering the same landmarks marked on the navigation module in the patient. The magnetic tracking guide is inserted through the bronchoscope, and at the procedure the same landmarks are marked, i.e. the main carina, the right upper lobe carina, the middle lobe carina, the left main carina and the carina between the left basal segments and the apical segment of the left lower lobe (Fig. 11.5). This is achieved by applying the magnetic locator guide at the carina and using a foot pedal to mark this point. The system then correlates the two pieces of data and co-registers the information.

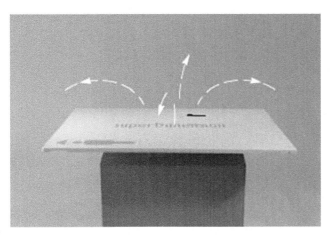
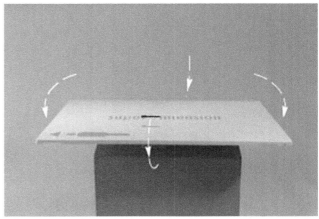

Fig. 11.4 *Electromagnetic board with the field depicted with white arrows and the locatable guide as a black arrow moving through the field.*

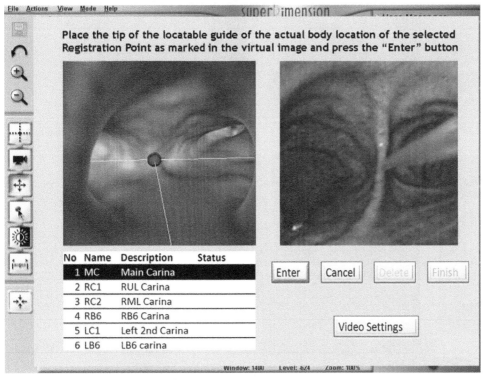

Fig. 11.5a *Registration process with the module showing virtual bronchoscopy and locatable guide on a real-time bronchoscopic image co-registering the following: the main carina (MC).*

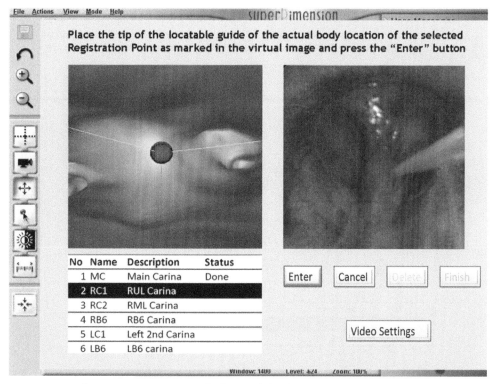

Fig. 11.5b *Registration process with the module showing virtual bronchoscopy and locatable guide on a real-time bronchoscopic image co-registering the following: the right upper lobe carina.*

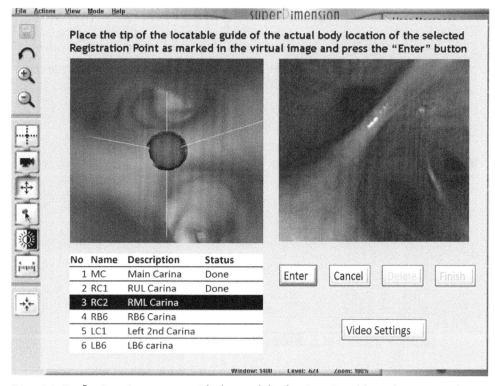

Fig. 11.5c *Registration process with the module showing virtual bronchoscopy and locatable guide on a real-time bronchoscopic image co-registering the following: the right middle lobe carina (RC2).*

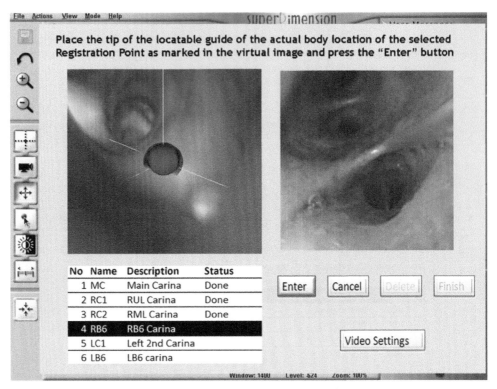

Fig. 11.5d *Registration process with the module showing virtual bronchoscopy and locatable guide on a real-time bronchoscopic image co-registering the following: the carina between the apical basal segment (RB6) and basal segments.*

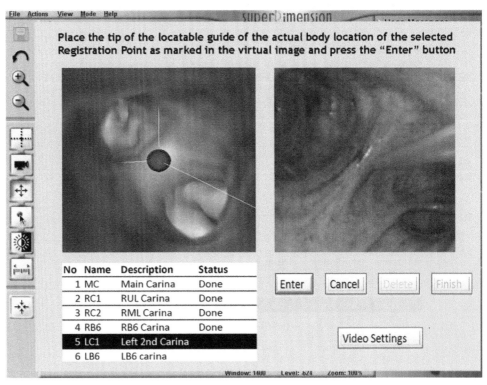

Fig. 11.5e *Registration process with the module showing virtual bronchoscopy and locatable guide on a real-time bronchoscopic image co-registering the following: the left secondary carina (LC1).*

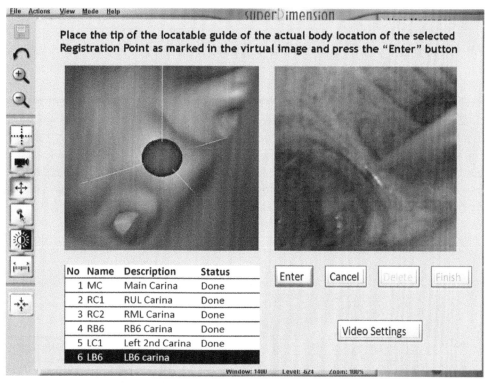

Place the tip of the locatable guide of the actual body location of the selected Registration Point as marked in the virtual image and press the "Enter" button

No	Name	Description	Status
1	MC	Main Carina	Done
2	RC1	RUL Carina	Done
3	RC2	RML Carina	Done
4	RB6	RB6 Carina	Done
5	LC1	Left 2nd Carina	Done
6	LB6	LB6 carina	

Fig. 11.5f *Registration process with the module showing virtual bronchoscopy and locatable guide on a real-time bronchoscopic image co-registering the following: the carina between the apical basal segment (LB6) and basal segments.*

The system calculates the error between the two pieces of data, i.e. computed tomography (CT) and patient data, and the lower the system error, the more accurate the navigation. The latest version of iLogic's software automatically co-registers the CT and patient data. The locatable guide is inserted through the instrument channel of the bronchoscope with the tip protruding. The bronchoscope is then navigated through the airways and during this process the system co-registers numerous data points, thus improving accuracy. The system also allows the manual registration process if required.

The locatable guide is manoeuvred to the target area using a steerable catheter (Fig. 11.6). This catheter moves in 12 different directions with a dial on its handle (akin to a clock face) that can be adjusted to different positions. The handle also allows varying amounts of pressure to change the degree of bend in the catheter.

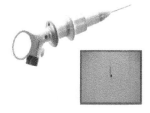

Fig. 11.6a *Movement of the steerable catheter in directions akin to a clock face: 12 o'clock direction (note the position of the red arrow on the catheter handle).*

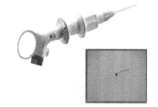

Fig. 11.6b *Movement of the steerable catheter in directions akin to a clock face: 2 o'clock direction.*

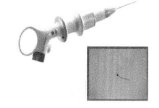

Fig. 11.6c *Movement of the steerable catheter in directions akin to a clock face: 4 o'clock direction.*

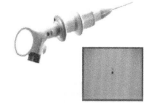

Fig. 11.6d *Movement of the steerable catheter in directions akin to a clock face: 11 o'clock direction (note the position of the red arrow on the catheter handle).*

Navigation

After inserting the catheter with the locatable guide to the appropriate bronchial segment, the navigation system can be used to guide it to the target location. The system shows the location of the guide on coronal, axial and sagittal CT sections (Fig. 11.7). There is also a screen which advises the operator in which direction, i.e. 1 o'clock or 2 o'clock etc., to manipulate the steerable catheter. A 'bull's eye' appears when the locatable guide is within 10 mm of the target location. Once the target is reached, the catheter is locked into position. The scope is held firmly in position, the locatable guide is removed and instruments such as cytology brushes, transbronchial needles and biopsy forceps can be passed through the steerable catheter in order to obtain samples from the target location. Where facilities exist, radial ultrasound probes or fluoroscopy can be used to verify the location of the catheter tip or locatable guide.

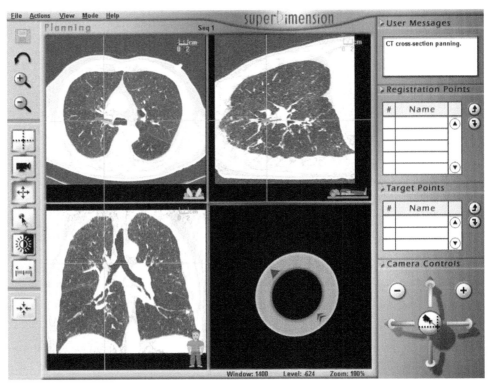

Fig. 11.7a *Navigation module showing the positions of the locatable guide on the CT sections (axial, sagittal and coronal) with a clock face guiding the manipulation of the steerable catheter: 10 o'clock position.*

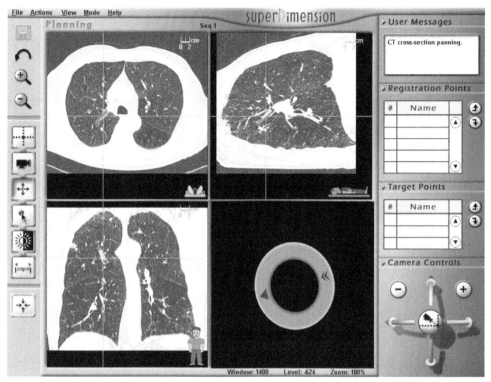

Fig. 11.7b *Navigation module showing the positions of the locatable guide on the CT sections (axial, sagittal and coronal) with a clock face guiding the manipulation of the steerable catheter: 8 o'clock position, guiding the catheter towards the right upper lobe.*

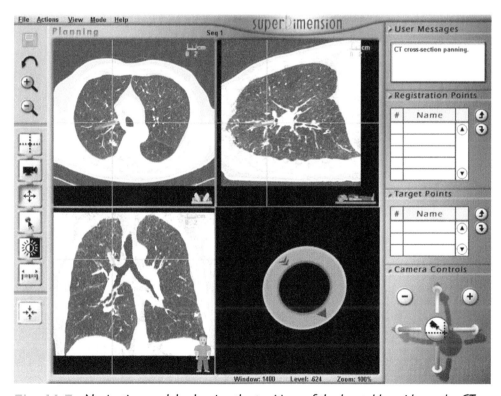

Fig. 11.7c *Navigation module showing the positions of the locatable guide on the CT sections (axial, sagittal and coronal) with a clock face guiding the manipulation of the steerable catheter: 5 o'clock position guiding the catheter towards the right upper lobe.*

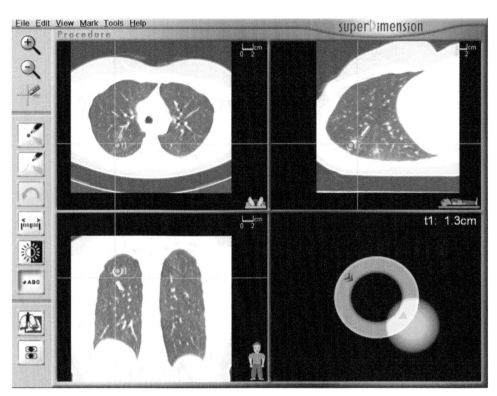

Fig. 11.7d *Navigation module showing the positions of the locatable guide on the CT sections (axial, sagittal and coronal) with a clock face guiding the manipulation of the steerable catheter: locatable guide close to the target site – the green dot appears close to the steering guide (orange circle).*

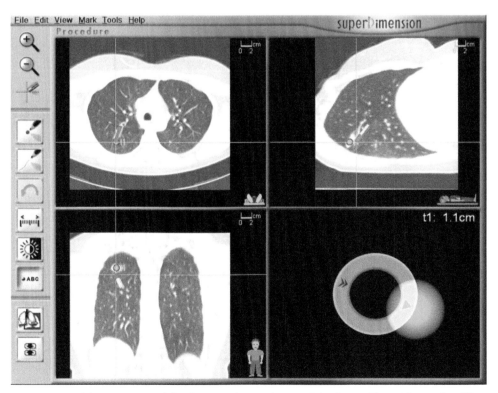

Fig. 11.7e *Navigation module showing the positions of the locatable guide on the CT sections (axial, sagittal and coronal) with a clock face guiding the manipulation of the steerable catheter: locatable guide within 11 mm of the target site as indicated by green dot being close to the steering guide.*

● Recent advances

With the latest iLogic™ software, the navigation module now has six possible screen modes. It creates a bronchial tree diagram with a route map to the target. After the registration process, the virtual bronchoscopy image displays the pathway to the target (Fig. 11.8). This facilitates navigation of the bronchoscope to the wedge position. From that point onwards the images can be set to display the clock face with CT sections to guide the steerable catheter to the target site. A close-up image can be selected when the locatable guide is within 10 mm of the target site to guide the optimal position for sampling.

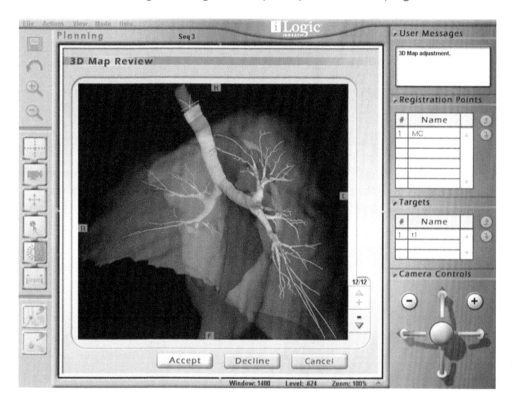

Fig. 11.8a *iLogic™ software module with three-dimensional bronchial tree.*

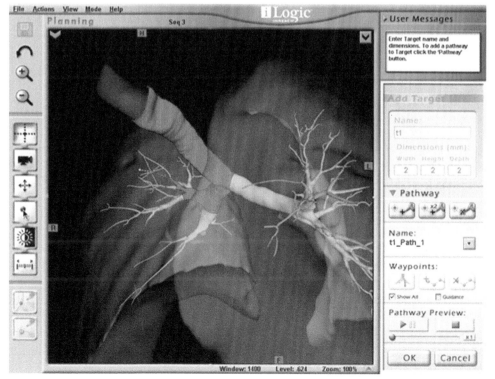

Fig. 11.8b *iLogic™ software with three-dimensional bronchial tree and route to the target highlighted in pink.*

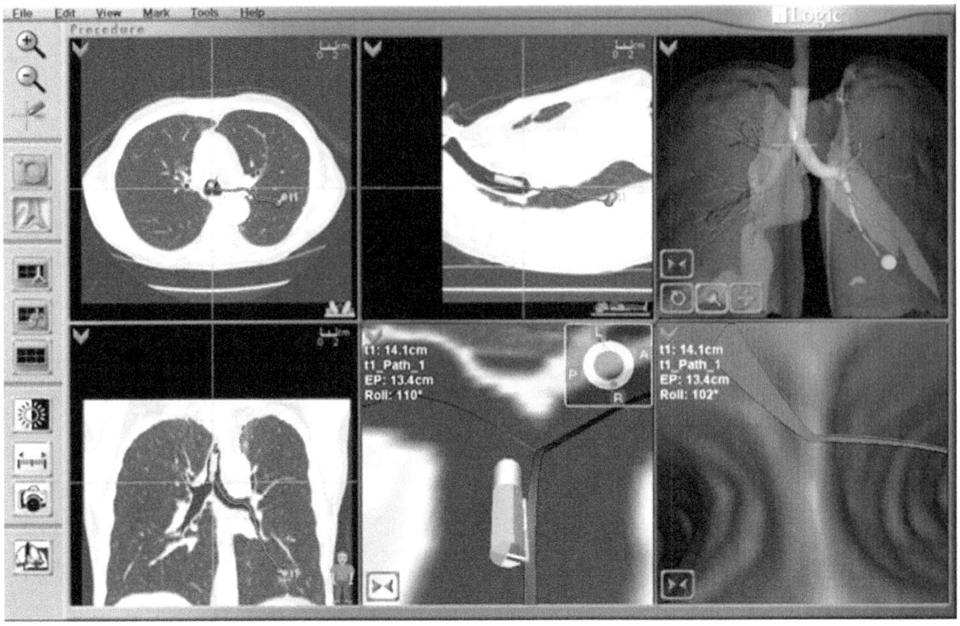

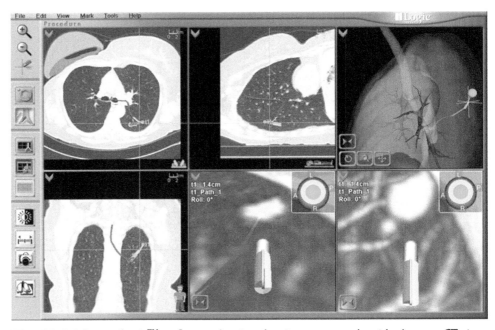

Fig. 11.8c *Latest iLogic™ software showing the six-screen mode with axial, coronal and sagittal CT views, with the position of the locatable guide and the virtual bronchoscopy with the route to the target.*

Fig. 11.8d *Latest iLogic™ software showing the six-screen mode with close-up CT views when the locatable guide is close to the target.*

For diagnostic purposes it may be more appropriate to set a target point where an airway is leading into the lesion. By contrast, a target area where the airway is passing lateral to the lesion may be closer but less likely to have a diagnostic yield. When inserting fiducial markers for radiotherapy or guides for video-assisted thoracoscopic biopsy, accurate positioning of the markers within the lesion is not necessary. Placement of fiducial markers in three different spatial locations within 10 mm of the nodule or target area is acceptable. The superDimension® navigation system can also be used to place a catheter in a more distal location for brachytherapy.

Intubation and management of airway haemorrhage

CHAPTER 12

Intubation

Airway control is a primary skill that should be acquired by the interventional bronchoscopist. As a safety precaution and to facilitate rapid, repeated insertion and removal of the bronchoscope, patients should be intubated prior to any interventional procedures such as tumour ablation or stent insertion. A size 8.5 or 9.0 uncuffed endotracheal tube is recommended in men and a size 8.0–8.5 tube in women. The endotracheal tube is cut to the appropriate length – usually to the oral markings on the endotracheal tube – and placed over the bronchoscope (Fig. 12.1).

An endotracheal tube with a Murphy eye may be useful in some circumstances. Depending on the position it may allow ventilation of the contralateral lung during interventional procedures. Furthermore, any debris or tumour fragments would then tend to fall back into the lung being treated and not into the contralateral lung.

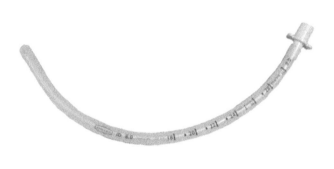

Fig. 12.1a *Uncuffed endotracheal tube (size 8.0, full length 32 cm).*

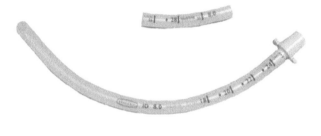

Fig. 12.1b *Endotracheal tube cut to marker for oral intubation (25 cm).*

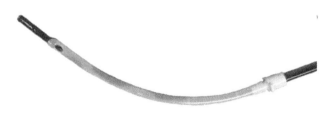

Fig. 12.1c *Uncuffed endotracheal tube with Murphy eye slid over the distal aspect of the bronchoscope.*

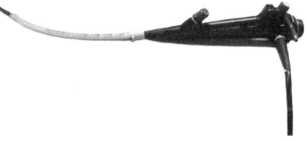

Fig. 12.1d *Uncuffed endotracheal tube slid over to the proximal aspect of the bronchoscope.*

An oral approach is preferred and the bronchoscope with an overlying endotracheal tube is inserted through a protective mouthpiece. Two or three 2 mL aliquots of 2 per cent lidocaine are applied to the vocal cords and the subglottic region. The bronchoscope is passed through the vocal cord and into the trachea. The patient is asked to take a deep breath and the endotracheal tube is then carefully slid over the bronchoscope and through the vocal cords. Small rotational movements are occasionally required while advancing the endotracheal tube.

The images in Figure 12.2 show the sequence of steps involved in intubation from topical application of lidocaine to the vocal cords through to insertion of the endotracheal tube through the vocal cords and into the trachea.

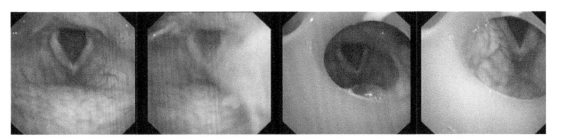

Fig. 12.2a *Sequence of images demonstrating intubation: topical lidocaine 2 per cent applied to the vocal cords. The endotracheal tube is moved to the distal aspect of the bronchoscope and over the vocal cords.*

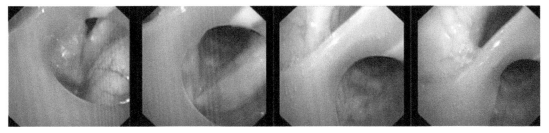

Fig. 12.2b *Sequence of images demonstrating intubation: uncuffed endotracheal tube inserted through the vocal cords and into the trachea.*

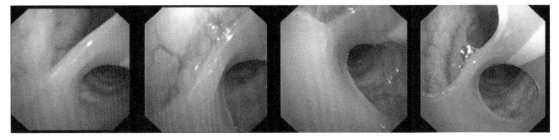

Fig. 12.2c *Sequence of images demonstrating intubation: endotracheal tube inserted into the trachea.*

In our experience, with adequate topical anaesthesia patients have tolerated an endotracheal tube for up to 1 hour with minimal conscious sedation (0–5 mg midazolam intravenously). The main caution is to avoid forcing the endotracheal tube against resistance, which is often due to the endotracheal tube being caught around the epiglottis or the vocal cords. Forceful insertion may lead to some trauma of the vocal cords (Fig. 12.3).

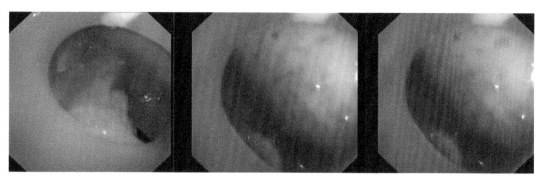

Fig. 12.3a *Sequence of images showing common problems with intubation: endotracheal tube caught on arytenoid cartilage.*

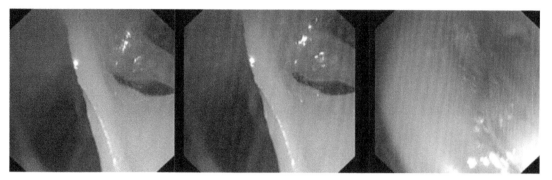

Fig. 12.3b *Sequence of images showing common problems with intubation: endotracheal tube caught on corniculate cartilage.*

Once the endotracheal tube is inserted, the assistant should hold the proximal portion in front of the patient's mouthpiece.

The key advantages of using an endotracheal tube is that it offers rapid and easy access into the airways, allowing the bronchoscope to be inserted and removed at will without causing any further inconvenience to the patient. This is particularly important for removing pieces of tumour during debulking and allows insertion of other accessories such as balloon blockers, which may be required in case of complications such as bleeding. It primarily allows safe airway management of the patient during interventional procedures.

A laryngeal mask is an alternative option to endotracheal intubation. Oxygenation during interventional procedures needs to be carefully managed. Hypoxia triggers cardiac arrhythmias and can increase the risk of complications. However, in certain procedures, such as laser treatment, the inspired oxygen (F_iO_2) should not be greater than 0.4. During such procedures, patients may need cyclical oxygen administration followed by short periods when the treatment is applied with a lower F_iO_2. We use a mask with a rebreather bag and cut out a piece on the side of the mask which allows access to the endotracheal tube and for the bronchoscope to pass in and out.

Balloon catheters

Balloon catheters are used for a number of purposes, including collapse of a lung during surgery. For our purpose, the primary aim is to enable airway control of massive haemorrhage.

● *Cohen endobronchial balloon blocker*

The Cohen endobronchial balloon blocker has a tip that can be deflected (Fig. 12.4). It can be inserted through an adaptor which attaches to the distal end of the endotracheal tube. The balloon catheter is inserted through the side-angled port of this adaptor and through the endotracheal tube into the right or left main bronchus. It naturally tends to go down the right main bronchus but can be manipulated or steered by a small degree in order to place the balloon in the left side. There is a gauge on the proximal end which, when turned, pulls on an in-built thread-wire and causes the distal tip of the catheter to bend (Fig. 12.5). The proximal and distal aspects of the catheter are marked with an arrow in the direction in which the tip tends to deflect. Therefore the blocker should be inserted through the endotracheal tube so that the arrows denoting direction of deflection are in the appropriate position.

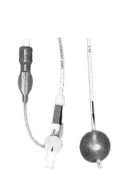 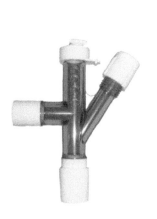 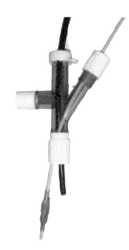

Fig. 12.4a *Cohen tip deflecting balloon catheter.*

Fig. 12.4b *Endotracheal tube mount adaptor for use with balloon catheters.*

Fig. 12.4c *Endotracheal tube mount adaptor with balloon catheter and bronchoscope in position.*

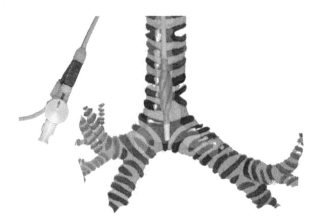 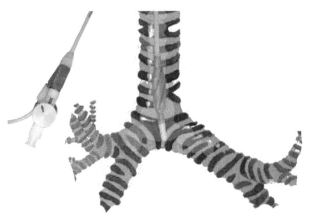

Fig. 12.5a *Cohen tip deflecting balloon catheter shown in various positions: neutral position.*

Fig. 12.5b *Cohen tip deflecting balloon catheter shown in various positions: dial moved by 45° anticlockwise causing a small deflection in the balloon tip.*

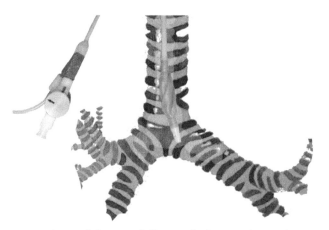

Fig. 12.5c *Cohen tip deflecting balloon catheter shown in various positions: dial moved by 90° anticlockwise causing a deflection in the balloon tip.*

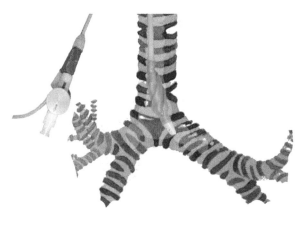

Fig. 12.5d *Cohen tip deflecting balloon catheter shown in various positions: dial moved by 180° anticlockwise causing further deflection in the balloon tip.*

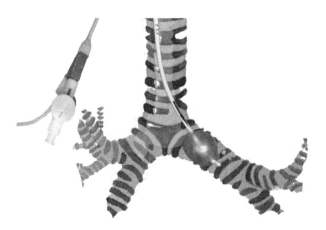

Fig. 12.5e *Cohen tip deflecting balloon catheter shown in various positions: inserted into the left main bronchus with the balloon inflated.*

Careful manipulation of the catheter and position of the patient's head allows the catheter to be introduced into the left main bronchus. This position is often the main bronchus but the balloon blocker may be advanced further into a lobar bronchus. The balloon can be inflated with about 4 mL of air. The exact amount should be checked in each patient prior to proceeding with the interventional aspect of the procedure. The catheter can be locked into position by tightening the screw fitting on the port of the endotracheal tube adaptor through which the blocker was introduced.

Insertion into the left main bronchus

The sequence of images in Figures 12.6 and 12.7 shows insertion of the balloon catheter into the left main bronchus. Occasionally the balloon catheter tip has a tendency to repeatedly go down the right side and then catch on the cartilage rings or carina, preventing correct placement. Figure 12.8 demonstrates this problem and also how it can be overcome by manipulation of the balloon tip and applying gentle torsion to the balloon catheter. Inflation of the balloon may also help when a balloon is partly inserted into the desired airway but stuck on a cartilage ring.

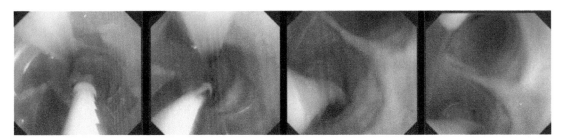

Fig. 12.6a *Sequences showing the insertion of a Cohen tip deflecting balloon catheter into the left main bronchus: inserted into the right main bronchus.*

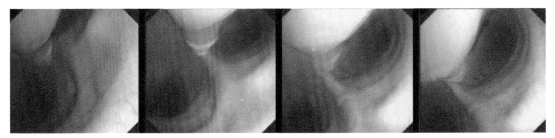

Fig. 12.6b *Sequences showing the insertion of a Cohen tip deflecting balloon catheter into the left main bronchus: being withdrawn from the right main bronchus to the carina and then being manipulated into the left main bronchus.*

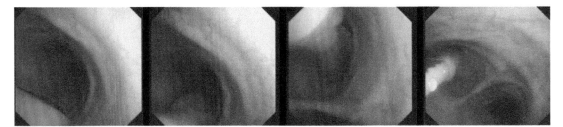

Fig. 12.6c *Sequences showing the insertion of a Cohen tip deflecting balloon catheter into the left main bronchus: being manipulated into the left main bronchus. Note the arrow at the tip of the catheter, which indicates the direction of deflection.*

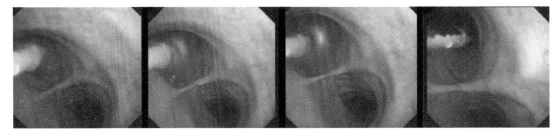

Fig. 12.6d *Sequences showing the insertion of a Cohen tip deflecting balloon catheter into the left main bronchus: positioned in the left main bronchus with balloon being inflated.*

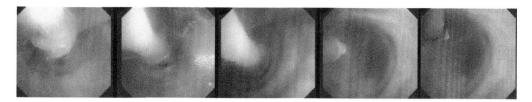

Fig. 12.7a *Cohen tip deflecting balloon catheter: being inserted via the endotracheal tube and into the lower trachea – the tip is directed into left main bronchus.*

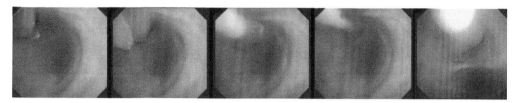

Fig. 12.7b *Cohen tip deflecting balloon catheter: in the left main bronchus.*

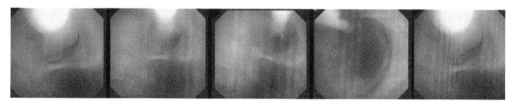

Fig. 12.7c *Cohen tip deflecting balloon catheter: in the left main bronchus with the balloon being inflated.*

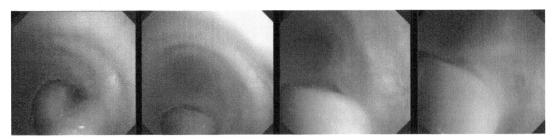

Fig. 12.8a *Sequence showing difficult insertion of the Cohen tip deflecting balloon catheter into the left main bronchus: the balloon catheter first enters the right main bronchus.*

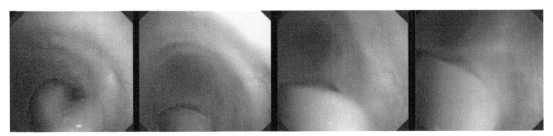

Fig. 12.8b *Sequence showing difficult insertion of the Cohen tip deflecting balloon catheter into the left main bronchus: the balloon catheter is withdrawn from the right main bronchus.*

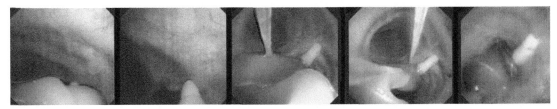

Fig. 12.8c *Sequence showing difficult insertion of the Cohen tip deflecting balloon catheter into the left main bronchus: the catheter tip is caught on the cartilage ring above the carina.*

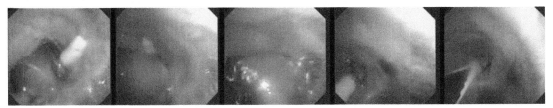

Fig. 12.8d *Sequence showing difficult insertion of the Cohen tip deflecting balloon catheter into the left main bronchus: the balloon catheter inserted in an inverted position into the left main bronchus. Balloon inflation is being attempted to try to push the tip down into the left main bronchus. The balloon is finally inserted down into the left main bronchus. The balloon is then inflated to check position.*

The series of images in Figure 12.9 shows the problems of overinflation or incorrect fixation of the balloon. This emphasizes the need to check placement by inflation of the balloon prior to commencing the interventional procedure.

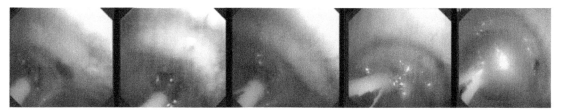

Fig. 12.9a *Sequence of images showing effects of inflating a balloon that is too proximal, with the tendency for the balloon to pop out of the left main bronchus.*

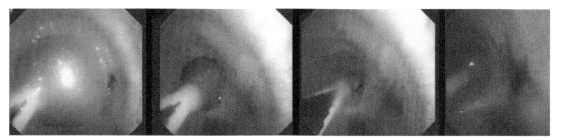

Fig. 12.9b *The problem is corrected by inserting the balloon further into the left main bronchus.*

In the event of significant haemorrhage or bleeding during the interventional procedure, the balloon can be inflated to isolate that lobe or side of the lung. This protects the contralateral lung from overspill of blood (which would affect its ventilation). The tamponade effect also helps to control the bleeding. The balloon is kept inflated for about 2 minutes and then carefully deflated. If fresh bleeding is still occurring, the balloon catheter should be inflated for a further 2-minute cycle.

● *Arndt endobronchial balloon blocker*

The Arndt endobronchial balloon blocker has a small adjustable loop at the end. This is designed to be used in conjunction with a small-calibre bronchoscope. The kit contains a multi-port adaptor which should be attached to the endotracheal tube (Fig. 12.10). The balloon should be fully deflated and the endobronchial blocker lubricated. It is inserted through the angled port which is designed for the blocker. The cap on this port can be screwed down to tighten the grip around the blocker and loosened to allow greater manipulation. The endobronchial blocker is advanced until it is visible in the mid-portion of the adaptor. The bronchoscope is then advanced through the central port and advanced through the loop on the endobronchial blocker. The loop is coupled to the bronchoscope by pulling back on the snare and can also be loosened by reducing the tension on the snare. Once the loop is tightened around the bronchoscope, the endobronchial blocker can be guided to any lobar bronchus (Fig. 12.11). Once in the correct position, the snare should be loosened and the bronchoscope can then be withdrawn leaving the balloon blocker in position.

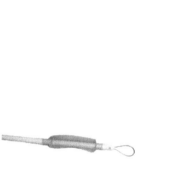

Fig. 12.10a *Arndt balloon catheter (note the loop on the distal tip).*

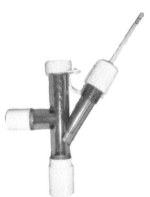

Fig. 12.10b *Arndt balloon catheter inserted through a multi-port adaptor.*

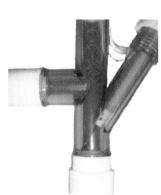

Fig. 12.10c *Arndt balloon catheter inserted through a mutli-port adaptor: note the position of the loop.*

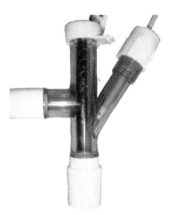

Fig. 12.10d *Bronchoscope and Arndt blocker inserted through the mutli-port adaptor.*

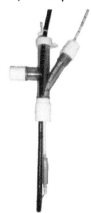

Fig. 12.10e *Arndt balloon catheter inserted through a mutli-port adaptor: bronchoscope passed through the loop at the distal end of the Arndt catheter.*

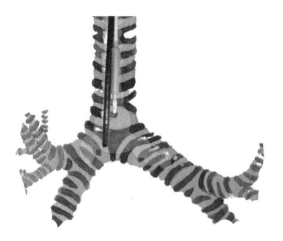

Fig. 12.11a *Arndt balloon catheter and bronchoscope: in neutral position in the trachea.*

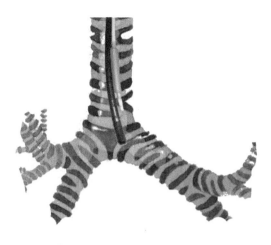

Fig. 12.11b *Arndt balloon catheter and bronchoscope: being directed into left main bronchus.*

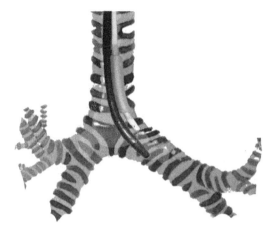

Fig. 12.11c *Arndt balloon catheter and bronchoscope: being directed into left main bronchus.*

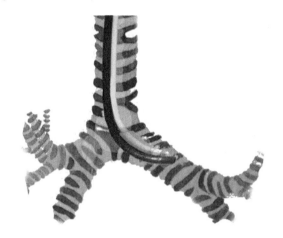

Fig. 12.11d *Arndt balloon catheter and bronchoscope: positioned in the left main bronchus.*

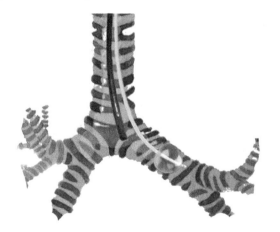

Fig. 12.11e *Arndt balloon catheter and bronchoscope: bronchoscope being withdrawn after positioning the Arndt balloon catheter in the left main bronchus and inflating it.*

Management of airway bleeding

Ice-cold saline, adrenaline (1 mL aliquots of 1:100 000) and balloon catheters should be available prior to any interventional procedure. In the event of bleeding, the first key principle is to remain calm and not to remove the bronchoscope from the airways. The scope should be moved more proximally from the source of bleeding and continued suction applied in order to maintain the airways free of blood. Suctioning a little way away from the source of bleeding also ensures that clot formation is not impaired. If the bleeding persists, inject a few mL of aliquots of ice-cold saline. Continue with regular suction in order to ensure optimal clearance of any blood which will otherwise affect ventilation. If this is unsuccessful and bleeding continues, instil 1–2 mL aliquots of 1:100 000 adrenaline. Follow this by effective suction of any blood that could clot and occlude adjacent airways (see the bleeding protocol in Box 12.1).

BOX 12.1 Bleeding protocol

Step 1
- Keep bronchoscope there
- Do not remove bronchoscope
  - Suction, suction, suction
  - Cold saline, cold saline
  - Suction
  - Adrenaline
  - Suction
  - Adrenaline
  - Call for help

Step 2
- Balloon blocker
- If Cohen blocker is ready in airway, deploy and inflate
- If not in place, use Arndt balloon blocker (couple with bronchoscope prior to insertion into the airways)
- Suction any blood in the airways especially in the contralateral lung
- Deflate balloon after 2 minutes and check if still bleeding
- If still bleeding, re-inflate and continue with proximal suctioning
- Ensure adequate ventilation of the patient
- Consider turning patient on to the side of bleeding

Key points
- A – suction, airway control
- B – ventilate through endotracheal tube with L-shaped adaptor
- C – Intravenous access, fluid, urgent cross-match blood, fresh frozen plasma
- D – Consider turning patient on to the side of bleeding

If the patient is intubated with an endotracheal tube, consider insertion of a balloon catheter; or if the balloon catheter is already in place prior to the interventional procedure, inflate the balloon and occlude the lobe or affected lung (Fig. 12.12). The balloon should be inflated for at least 2 minutes. During this period any blood that has spilled into the contralateral lung should be suctioned away to ensure optimal ventilation. After 2 minutes the balloon is deflated slowly. Suction is maintained to clear any residual blood, but care must be taken not to dislodge or clear any clot that has been formed around the site of bleeding. If there is still persistent bleeding then the balloon should be reinflated for a further 2-minute cycle. The patient can also be turned on to the side of bleeding to enhance the tamponade effect and allow maximal activity of the unaffected lung.

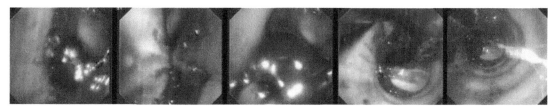

Fig. 12.12a *Active brisk bleeding from right lower lobe managed with a cycle of suction, ice-cold saline and dilute adrenaline. The Cohen balloon blocker is inflated to isolate the right lung.*

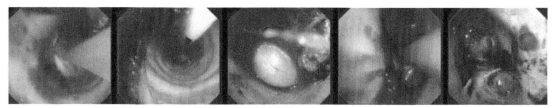

Fig. 12.12b *Cohen balloon blocker inflated to isolate right lung with suction of blood from the remaining airways. The balloon is deflated after 2 minutes. Saline is instilled and gentle suction is applied proximally in the right lower lobe after deflation and removal of the Cohen balloon.*

In the situation where there is spontaneous massive bleeding and no endotracheal tube is in place, it is important to retain the bronchoscope in position and maintain suction. Where skills exist, an attempt should be made to intubate the patient either via standard laryngoscope or by sleeving it over the bronchoscope and then under direct vision. An alternative is to use the video laryngoscope. This should be done as quickly and efficiently as possible immediately after intubation; any blood that has spilled into the normal side should be suctioned and cleared first.

The easiest balloon to use is the Arndt balloon. The balloon catheter is inserted through the endotracheal tube, and biopsy or grasping forceps are introduced through the working channel of the bronchoscope. The forceps are then used to grasp the balloon and the balloon can then be directed towards the lobar bronchus, from where the bleeding is originating. The balloon is then inserted to tamponade the bleeding for at least 2–3 minutes. With practice this technique can be utilized very quickly and effectively.

Alternatively the multi-port adaptor can be set up with the Arndt balloon blocker and bronchoscope. Once the loop is coupled with the bronchoscope, the unit can be attached to the endotracheal tube and manipulated to the target lobe in the patient. In the emergency situation, it is quicker to simply occlude the lung where the bleeding is originating. Mortality and morbidity from airway haemorrhage are usually due to loss of gas exchange as a result of the blood clotting off the airways before exsanguination becomes a factor. Hence, if you block off the lung which is the source of the haemorrhage then you protect the other lung from overspill of blood and consequent occlusion of the airways. Suctioning of any blood that has spilled over into the normal side helps to maximize oxygenation of the patient.

CHAPTER 13

Endobronchial tumour debulking

Central airway tumours cause significant morbidity and mortality. The effects include airflow obstruction with dyspnoea, haemoptysis, impaired clearance of secretions with repeated infections and pneumonia. In patients who are inoperable due to advanced disease or significant comorbidity, active palliation by debulking the endobronchial tumour is an important aspect of treatment. Although there are no definitive randomized control trials, tumour ablation by a variety of techniques has been shown to improve dyspnoea, reduce frequency of haemoptysis, improve quality of life and potentially improve survival.

A variety of techniques are available for tumour debulking and the choice is dependent on local availability and expertise. All the available techniques are of similar efficacy. Electrocautery or diathermy tends to be available in most endoscopy units and is relatively inexpensive. Similarly, cryotherapy equipment is inexpensive compared to the neodymium-yttrium aluminium garnet (Nd-Yag) laser which has much higher capital and maintenance costs. We predominantly use electrocautery and a modified version of cryotherapy termed cryoextraction – these are the main focus of this chapter.

Electrocautery

Electrocautery or diathermy is an alternative technique for tumour ablation. It utilizes high-frequency alternating current (10-5 to 10-7 Hz) to generate heat locally and induce coagulation and tissue necrosis. Low-frequency current stimulates nerves and muscle fibres and is therefore not used. The resistance within a tissue where the electrical current is applied leads to the generation of heat. Diathermy or electrocautery requires the use of special insulated flexible bronchoscopes. The patient plate is required to ground the patient and hence complete the circuit. This should be a large surface such as the back of the thigh in order to easily conduct electricity away. Poor conduction around the patient plate would also lead to heat generation and local burns.

Electrocautery is performed with a number of accessories, such as a coagulation probe, snares, biopsy forceps and a cutting knife (Fig. 13.1).

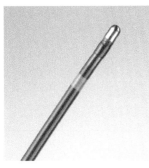

Fig. 13.1a *Electrocautery accessories: coagulation probe.*

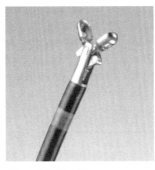

Fig. 13.1b *Electrocautery accessories: hot biopsy forceps.*

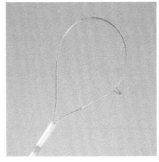

Fig. 13.1c *Electrocautery accessories: snare.*

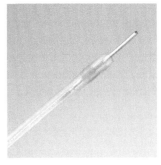

Fig. 13.1d *Electrocautery accessories: electrosurgical knife.*

Low-voltage, high-amperage current leads to coagulation, whereas cutting involves high voltage and low amperage. A blend of these two modes is used to achieve tissue destruction with coagulation. Electrocautery allows rapid ablation of the tumour and restoration of airway patency. Hence, electrocautery can be used in an acute setting where rapid restoration of airway patency is required. A coagulation probe is a blunt probe and is usually the first tool used (Fig. 13.2). A test patch on normal mucosa derives some information and allows the power setting to be adjusted so that a small white blanched area is obtained on application of the electrocautery probe (usually 10–30 watts). Contact with the tumour with a 3–5 second activation should also provide some information about tumour susceptibility, friability and potential bleeding risk. Elongated or plaque-like lesions are amenable to treatment with a coagulation probe. It may also be used to free up tumour from edges of the airway wall.

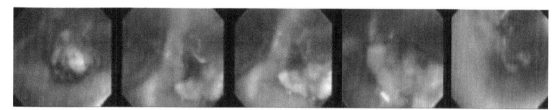

Fig. 13.2a *Coagulation probe and tumour visible in the left main bronchus. Note the green band protruding from the bronchoscope. The coagulation probe is inserted into the centre of the tumour.*

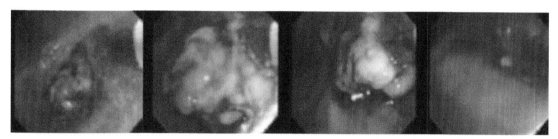

Fig. 13.2b *The edge of the tumour being treated with the coagulation probe in order to free the tumour from the airway. The coagulation probe is being used to free the lateral edge of the tumour and then the superior margin.*

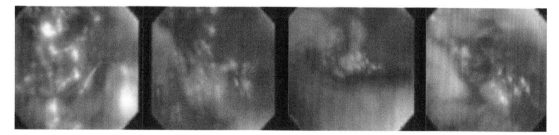

Fig. 13.2c *The coagulation probe is activated in a blend mode (combination of coagulation and cut) and moved from side to side to free the tumour from the airway wall. There is some debulking of tumour with the distal airway visible in the superolateral aspect.*

The electrosurgical snare is more effective in treating and removing polypoid lesions (Fig. 13.3). The snare is used to loop over the tissue and is then slowly tightened. The diathermy is activated as the snare is slowly tightened to cut and coagulate the tissue at the base. If the snare is tightened too quickly with inadequate electrocautery activation, the mechanical cheese-wire effect will cut off the tumour but without the coagulation effect and hence there is a greater risk of bleeding. After snaring the tissue, the bronchoscope with suction is applied to the free piece and the whole unit is removed via the endotracheal tube. Regular suction of blood debris is required. Good control of bleeding is necessary as it also impairs the effectiveness of electrocautery as the electricity is conducted over a much wider area and hence the local heating effect is significantly reduced.

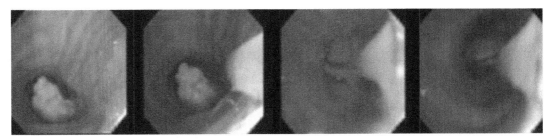

Fig. 13.3a *Electrosurgical snare placed around polypoid tumour originating from the left main bronchus into the trachea.*

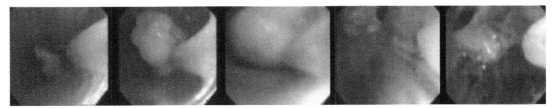

Fig. 13.3b *Once the snare is around tumour, the electrocautery is activated in 2-second bursts while the snare is slowly tightened around the tumour. The snare cuts through the tumour and is removed.*

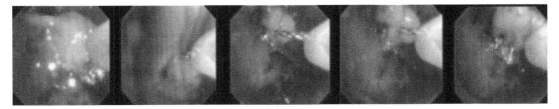

Fig. 13.3c *Snare opened and looped over residual tumour.*

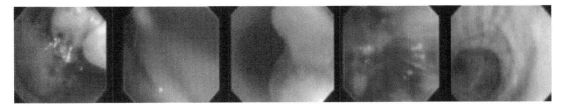

Fig. 13.3d *Resected tumour being withdrawn through the endotracheal tube with the bronchoscopic view from the trachea showing complete resection of tumour from the left main bronchus.*

The hot biopsy forceps can also be used to debulk tumours. The forceps are used to bite on the tumour and are then gently pulled up prior to activating the diathermy energy. Electrical current accumulates at the base of the neck, heating that area and allowing a larger biopsied piece to be obtained with minimal bleeding.

The electrosurgical knife is sparingly used but is invaluable for treating tracheal and endobronchial webs. A cruciate incision can be performed on the web. Precautions when using electrocautery and its potential complications are shown in Boxes 13.1 and 13.2.

BOX 13.1 Precautions when performing electrocautery

- Ensure good contact of grounding plate on the patient
- Use insulated and (approved) bronchoscopes for electrocautery
- Remove rings or any pieces of metal on the patient
- Check with the cardiologist before treating patients with a pacemaker or implantable defibrillator
- Ensure $F_iO_2 < 0.4$ and in practical terms limit the gas flow to < 4 L/min via nasal cannulae (there is a risk of airway fire with high oxygen levels)
- Always ensure the green band on the electrocautery accessory (probe, snare etc.) is visible before activation of the diathermy unit

BOX 13.2 Complications of electrocautery

- Bleeding/haemorrhage
- Respiratory failure
- Tracheal or bronchial perforation
- Airway fire
- Pneumothorax
- Arrhythmias
- Post-treatment stenosis
- Pneumonia

Argon plasma coagulation

Argon plasma coagulation is a non-contact form of electrocautery (Fig. 13.4). Ionized argon gas is created by a high-frequency generator and flows through a Teflon catheter. A wire within the catheter conducts the high-frequency current and a tungsten tip at the end converts the argon to an ionized plasma. The electricity is conducted through the gas plasma. It is very effective at coagulation and has a fixed depth of penetration of 3–5 mm. The rapid coagulating effect is very useful at treating the surface of exophytic tumours that are bleeding. The plasma also tends to bend to the part of least resistance and can be used to treat areas that are not accessible to conventional electrocautery coagulation probes. Both end-firing and side-firing treatment catheters are available. The argon flow is typically set between 0.3 and 2.0 L/min with the wattage at 30 to 40 W.

The precautions when using argon plasma coagulation and its complications are similar to those of electrocautery.

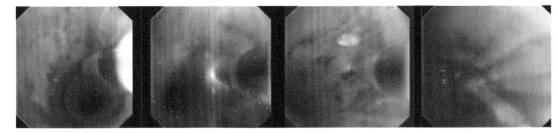

Fig. 13.4a *Argon plasma coagulation activated in the airway. Note that the first black marking band is visible, indicating that the catheter is a safe distance from the tip of the bronchoscope. A test area of coagulation is performed in the airway to check the energy level selected.*

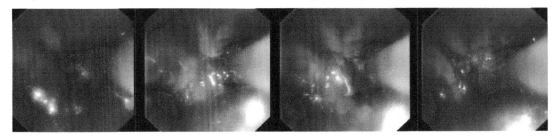

Fig. 13.4b *Argon plasma coagulation of the vascular right middle lobe tumour.*

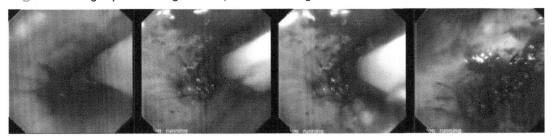

Fig. 13.4c *Vascular right middle lobe tumour treated with spray coagulation to the surface. The whole surface of tumour in the right middle lobe is coagulated.*

Cryotherapy

Obstructing endobronchial tumours can be easily relieved with cryotherapy extraction of the tumours. Cryotherapy can be used in its traditional format or by cryoextraction.

Traditional cryotherapy involves the application of the cryoprobe directly on to the tumour (Fig. 13.5). The cryoprobe itself is passed through the instrument channel, until the tip protrudes by about 2 cm from the distal end of the bronchoscope. The probes are marked and hence should be advanced until a clear distal black band is visible on the probe. This is to prevent accidental freezing and damage of the bronchoscope. Under direct vision, the probe is applied to the tumour and the freezing process is activated with a foot pedal and the tissue frozen for approximately 10 seconds depending on the constitution of the tumour. The extent of tissue that is frozen can be visually identified by the ice-front. The tissue is then allowed to thaw and further freeze cycles are applied. Multiple overlapping applications are performed to ensure that the whole endobronchial tumour is adequately treated.

The freezing leads to vasoconstriction and microthrombi formation, which in turn reduce the blood supply to the tumour. Freezing also leads to protein and enzyme damage and the net effect is cell necrosis. Mechanical damage from the formation of ice crystals may also explain some of the necrosis. Repeated freeze–thaw cycles lead to overall tumour necrosis. This technique is easily and safely applied, but the main disadvantage is its delayed effect. A repeat bronchoscopy is usually required 72 hours to 1 week after the initial procedure to remove the necrotic tumour debris. Hence it is not an appropriate technique in the presence of a critical lesion.

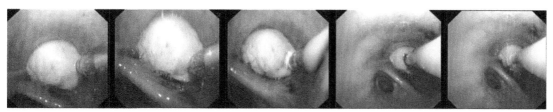

Fig. 13.5a *Cryoprobe activated while in contact with tumour and with an ice ball formed around the tip of the cryoprobe.*

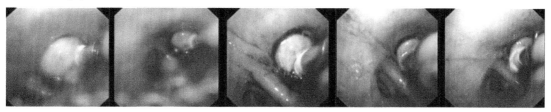

Fig. 13.5b *The probe is allowed to thaw and then the cryoprobe is moved a few mm to the side and activated again.*

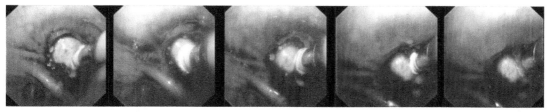

Fig. 13.5c *Note the formation of the ice-front around the tip of the probe. The ice-front enlarges with continued application of the cryoprobe. Regression of the ice-front is observed after switching off the probe.*

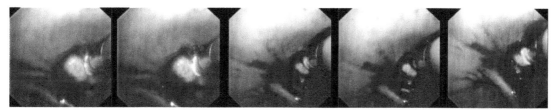

Fig. 13.5d *The cryoprobe again moved a few mm and activated to create multiple overlapping areas of treatment.*

● Cryoextraction

Cryoextraction utilizes a modified cryoprobe from Erbe where the central gas channel has been stabilized and the joint between the probe and the catheter is strengthened to withstand forces of up to 50 newtons. The cryoprobe is cooled down to temperatures of around − 90°C at the tip of the probe on activation and freezes tissue in contact with the probe (Fig. 13.6). The probe is applied to the tumour and activated for about 3–6 seconds. The duration is modulated according to the size of the ice-front and the tissue being treated. The bronchoscope and probe are gently tugged together as one unit and a piece of tumour adhering to the probe is extracted. The bronchoscope and probe are removed via the endotracheal tube, the tissue is allowed to thaw and is then removed from the probe. The bronchoscope and probe are then re-inserted through the endotracheal tube and another piece of tumour frozen with the cryoprobe and extracted. With this technique, airway obstruction from tumours can be quickly and effectively debulked to alleviate airway obstruction.

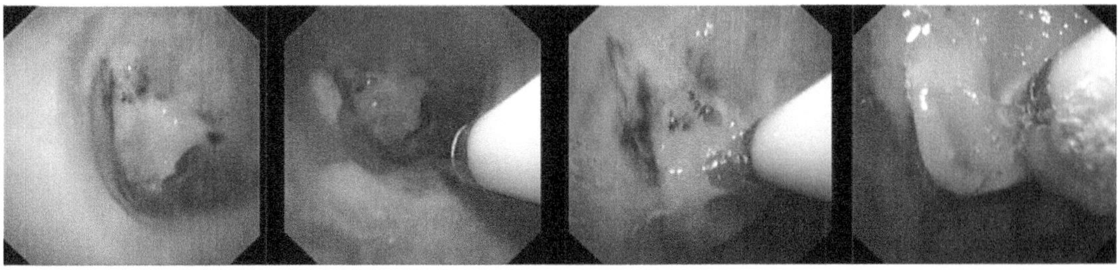

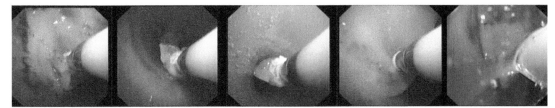

Fig. 13.6a *Necrotic tumour almost completely occluding the right main bronchus. The cryoprobe is activated after contact with the tumour.*

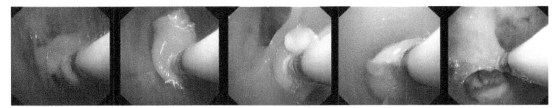

Fig. 13.6b *The tumour adheres to the tip of the cryoprobe and the adherent tumour is broken off. The cryoprobe with adherent tumour and bronchoscope are removed as one unit via the endotracheal tube.*

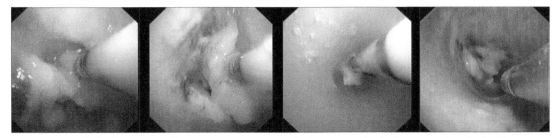

Fig. 13.6c *Ice-front formed in the tumour in the area of contact with the cryoprobe. The adherent tumour is being gently pulled to detach another piece of tumour.*

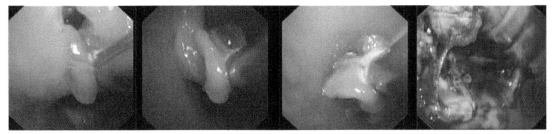

Fig. 13.6d *A further piece of tumour in contact with the cryoprobe is frozen and pulled off.*

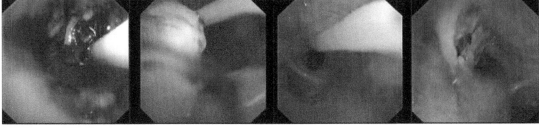

Fig. 13.6e *Significant debulking of the tumour with cyclical freezing and breaking off adherent frozen tumour.*

Fig. 13.6f *Restoration of patency in the right main bronchus with pus arising through the reopened airway.*

Laser treatment

Neodymium–yttrium aluminium garnet laser is usually used through a rigid bronchoscope but flexible fibres are also available which can be used through a flexible bronchoscope. This laser tends to vaporize tissue. The power should be limited to 40 watts as the depth of penetration can vary according to the tissue composition and clinical trials have shown an increased frequency of adverse events in power settings above 40 watts. The colour of the tissue may also affect the thermal energy absorbed.

The laser is delivered through flexible fibres, but the laser light itself is invisible (wavelength = 1064 nanometres) and hence is used in conjunction with red helium-neon aiming beam to guide treatment application. The precautions to be taken when using laser are shown in Box 13.3.

BOX 13.3 Precautions when using laser

- Inspired oxygen concentration (F_iO_2) < 0.4
- Limit power to less than 40 watts
- Protect the patient's eyes
- Ensure all personnel wear protective goggles
- Avoid its use in the presence of silicone or covered stents
- Ensure the distal tip is sufficiently beyond the tip of the bronchoscope

---

Photodynamic therapy

Photodynamic therapy utilizes a photosensitizer which is activated by a special light source. Photofrin is a commonly used agent that is administered 48 hours before the therapeutic bronchoscopy (dose 2 mg/kg intravenously). The drug is cleared from most tissues within 3 days but is retained in tumour tissue, skin, liver and spleen for up to 6 weeks. At bronchoscopy a non-thermal laser light such as potassium titanyl phosphate (KTP) or argon pumped laser is applied using a cylindrical diffuser. The laser light (wavelength 630 nanometres) penetrates the tissue and causes tumour destruction. The cylindrical diffuser tip is available in a variety of lengths and is chosen according to the tumour extent. The cylindrical diffuser is positioned adjacent to the tumour and the light is emitted in a 360° arc from the diffuser. Approximately 200 joules is applied per cm treated and this takes approximately 8 minutes. It is crucial to ensure that the tip is held in a stable position. If an untreated section is left, the diffuser can be repositioned and the additional area retreated. A repeat bronchoscopy should be performed after 48 hours to debulk any necrotic tissue and suction out any inflammatory debris and mucus.

The key complications are haemorrhage, hypoxia due to plugging of the airways, infection due to retention of secretions, and necrotic debris. The main side effect limiting the utility of photodynamic therapy is skin sensitivity. Retention of the photosensitizer in the skin means that exposure to light leads to burns. Patients are asked to completely cover their body and not expose themselves to light for at least 6 weeks. Late complications include circumferential strictures in the treated areas.

Brachytherapy

Brachytherapy involves the placement of a blind-ending catheter close to the tumour. Bronchoscopy with the nasal approach is performed and a polyethylene catheter is placed through the instrument channel of the bronchoscope and into the desired airway.

The catheter position can be verified with fluoroscopy if required. The bronchoscope is slowly withdrawn while the catheter is advanced. The catheter is secured in position at the nose and the bronchoscope is reintroduced through the oral route to check correct placement of the catheter.

The treatment area is planned using available radiology and the post-procedure chest radiograph. The treatment is performed in a lead-shielded room. A remote after-loading device is connected to the proximal portion of the catheter. According to the treatment area planned, the catheter is loaded with a combination of inactive and radioactive beads. High-dose brachytherapy is more commonly performed and uses an iridium-192 source.

The key complications of high-dose brachytherapy include massive haemoptysis, fistula formation, radiation bronchitis and stenosis. These risks are increased by concurrent external beam radiotherapy, previous endobronchial laser treatment, increasing dose intensity of brachytherapy and a cell subtype of large cell carcinoma.

Stents

Endobronchial or endotracheal stents are used where airway obstruction is caused by extrinsic compression from a tumour. They may also be required after endobronchial tumour debulking if the airway has lost its support structure and also if the tumour is prolapsing through a lobar bronchus and occluding the main bronchus. A variety of different stents exist, but the main group are metallic or non-metallic stents. Metallic stents themselves are subdivided into covered and uncovered stents. Non-metallic stents usually require insertion with a rigid bronchoscope and are not discussed further here. Metallic stents are usually made from nitinol (a nickel titanium alloy) (Fig. 14.1).

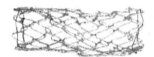

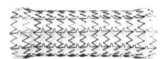

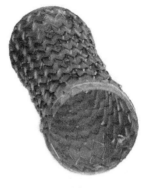

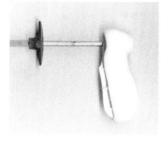

Fig. 14.1a *Self-expanding uncovered nitinol stent.*

Fig. 14.1b *Nitinol stent, laser-cut from a single piece and covered with silicon.*

Fig. 14.1c *Nitinol stent, laser-cut from a single piece and covered with silicon.*

Fig. 14.1d *Deployment handle for self-expanding stent.*

Technique of stent insertion

● *Direct vision*

The first step is to intubate the patient with a size 8 or 9 uncuffed endotracheal tube. An ultra-fine bronchoscope with an external diameter of 2.8 mm is used and the area of narrowing inspected under direct vision. A pulmonary guidewire (jagwire with a soft distal tip) is inserted through the instrument channel and passed through the stenotic airway into the distal aspects of the lung (Fig. 14.2). A wire exchange technique is employed in order to remove the bronchoscope while maintaining the jagwire in its current position. This is best achieved by feeding the wire a couple of centimetres deeper while removing the bronchoscope by a similar amount. This is performed until the bronchoscope is removed but the wire is maintained in position. The bronchoscope is passed through the endotracheal tube to check that the guidewire is still in the correct position. The guidewire should be held taut by an assistant and care taken to maintain its position,

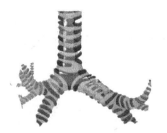

Fig. 14.2a *Narrowing in right main bronchus secondary to tumour.*

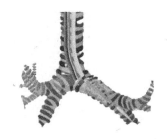

Fig. 14.2b *Guidewire inserted through a narrowed right main bronchial tumour.*

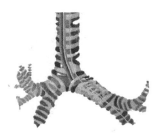

Fig. 14.2c *Bronchoscope removed while retaining guidewire in position through the right main bronchial tumour. The bronchoscope is then reinserted into the airway to check the position.*

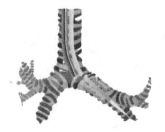

Fig. 14.2d *Stent inserted over the guidewire. The positioning of the stent is confirmed by bronchoscopy.*

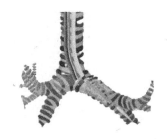

Fig. 14.2e *Initial deployment of the stent under bronchoscopic control.*

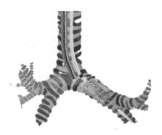

Fig. 14.2f *Gradual deployment of the stent under bronchoscopic control.*

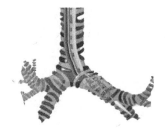

Fig. 14.2g *Full deployment of the stent under bronchoscopic control.*

The patient is then re-bronchoscoped by inserting the bronchoscope through the vocal cords via the oral route adjacent to the endotracheal tube. This allows the stent to be passed through the endotracheal tube and manipulated in the trachea or bronchi while maintaining vision with the bronchoscope (Fig. 14.3). The stent is fed over the guidewire through the endotracheal tube and into the desired location in the airways. The stents have markers highlighting the proximal end of the stent within the delivery catheter. Before the procedure, a CT scan of the thorax should be carefully studied to ensure that stenting is a suitable treatment option. For example, it is important to ascertain that there is a good patency of the airways beyond the stenosis. The size and length of the stents required can also be determined by the CT scan. This is complemented by careful examination of the airways at bronchoscopy.

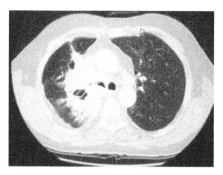

Fig. 14.3a *CT scan showing narrowing of the right main bronchus.*

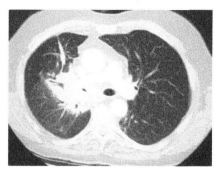

Fig. 14.3b *Concentric narrowing of the right main bronchus.*

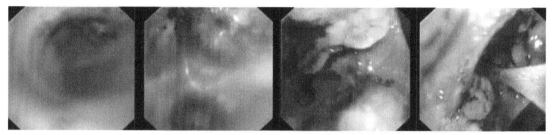

Fig. 14.3c *Concentric infiltration and narrowing of the right main bronchus. Guidewire inserted into the right main bronchus.*

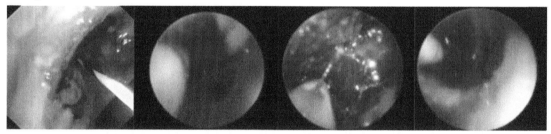

Fig. 14.3d *Guidewire advanced distally into the right main bronchus while sequentially withdrawing the bronchoscope. Delivery catheter with the stent advanced over the guidewire under bronchoscopic vision with 2.8 mm hybrid fibrescope (round images).*

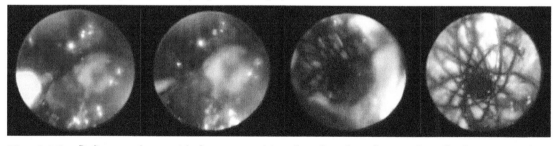

Fig. 14.3e *Delivery catheter with the stent positioned so that the yellow markers for the proximal limits of the stent are above the area of stenosis. Distal and proximal aspects of the stent are inspected.*

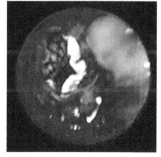

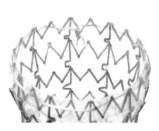

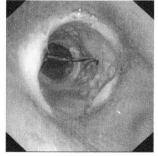

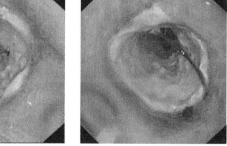

Fig. 14.3f *Stent placed in the constricted right main bronchus.*

Fig. 14.3g *Silicon-coated nitinol stent with a suture in the proximal aspect.*

Fig. 14.3h, i *Covered nitinol stent in the airway with a proximal silk thread which can be used to grab the stent and manipulate it into a more proximal position (the stent should not be pushed distally).*

The stent is carefully positioned so that the proximal marker is visible proximal to the area of narrowing under direct vision and the stent is carefully deployed. A variety of deployment mechanisms exist and in principle all use the technique of withdrawing the overlying protective catheter (Figs 14.4 and 14.5). Please check and familiarize yourself with the manufacturer's instructions. We recommend fixing the position of your arm, for example, holding the elbow fixed over your abdomen and then pulling back the overlying sheath over the stent. This is an important step for correct placement as there is a tendency to push forward during deployment and this leads to the stent being deployed further into the airways than desired. The stent should be deployed in a steady manner under direct vision so that any small adjustments can be made to ensure that the stent is optimally positioned prior to full deployment.

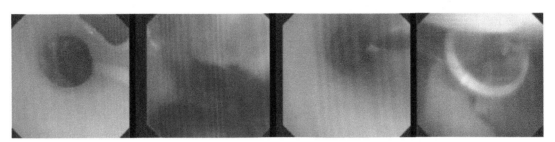

Fig. 14.4a *Following intubation, the guidewire is inserted into the narrowed right main bronchus.*

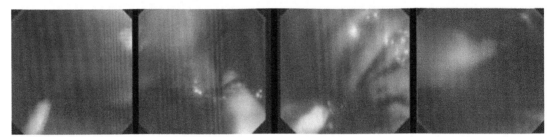

Fig. 14.4b *The stent is inserted through the narrowed right main bronchus and gradually deployed by removing the silk thread around the stent.*

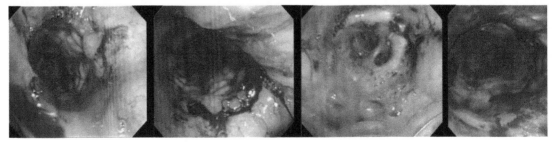

Fig. 14.4c *An uncovered nitinol stent which has been fully deployed with an improvement in the calibre of the right main bronchus.*

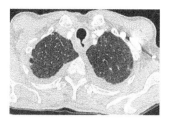

Fig. 14.5a *CT scan at the level of a tracheo-oesophageal fistula.*

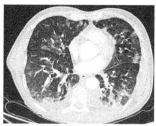

Fig. 14.5b *CT scan showing some changes of basal pneumonia due to aspiration.*

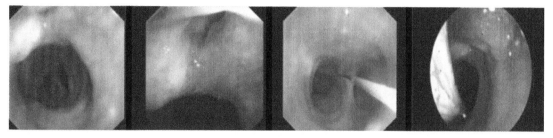

Fig. 14.5c *Tracheo-oesophageal fistula visible in the posterior aspect of the upper trachea. Stent inserted over the guidewire under visual control with a thin hybrid bronchoscope.*

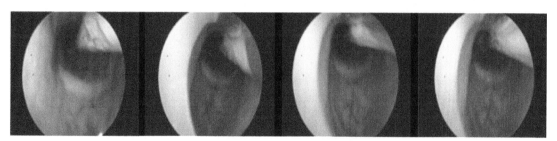

Fig. 14.5d *Covered nitinol stent being positioned in the trachea. The yellow marker defines the proximal limit of the stent and the stent is carefully positioned in the trachea to fully seal the tracheo-oesophageal fistula.*

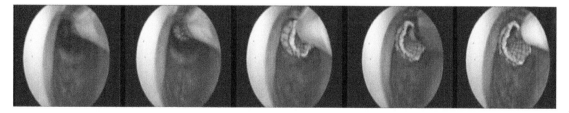

Fig. 14.5e *Steady deployment of stent in the trachea with repositioning of the stent in order to ensure an adequate seal of the tracheo-oesophageal fistula.*

Some of the stents can be manipulated into a proximal position by grasping a silk stitch at the end of the proximal portion of the stent with forceps and then gently moving the stent proximally (Fig. 14.3h,i). However, manipulating the stent by a precise amount is difficult and the stent should never be pushed distally.

● *Radiology-guided stent insertion*

Endotracheal and endobronchial stents can also be positioned and deployed under fluoroscopic guidance (Figs. 14.6 and 14.7). The initial steps are similar to deployment of the stents under direct vision. Once the guidewire is placed through the appropriate narrowed lobar bronchus, the stent is fed over the guidewire and through the endotracheal tube. Under fluoroscopic guidance the stent is advanced and positioned over the desired area. The stents usually have proximal and distal radiological markers, which allow the accurate positioning of the stent under fluoroscopic control. The deployment of the stent is again the same as with direct vision except on this occasion the fluoroscopy provides the visual guidance. Stents can also be placed with a combination of direct visual guidance and fluoroscopy. This may be more appropriate in circumstances where the distal aspect cannot be visualized at bronchoscopy even with an ultra-fine bronchoscope.

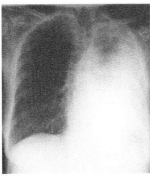

Fig. 14.6a *Chest radiograph of a patient with left lower lobe and lingular collapse.*

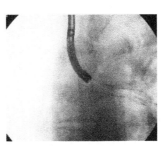

Fig. 14.6b *Stent positioned and deployed under fluoroscopic control.*

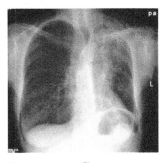

Fig. 14.6c *Chest radiograph showing significant reinflation of the left lung after stent placement (visible in the left main bronchus).*

Fig. 14.7a *Three silicon-coated stents inserted in a patient: one in the main carina with two other stents visible distally in the right and left main bronchi.*

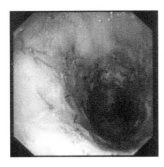

Fig. 14.7b *Close-up of the carina showing two stents from each main bronchus joining at the carina.*

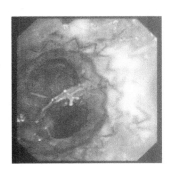

Complications of stents

Malignant endobronchial tumour involvement is the most common indication for tracheal or bronchial stents. Hence the covered variety is more frequently utilized. However, these stents impair normal mucociliary clearance and hence are prone to complications such as mucus retention and bio-fouling of the stents. This is where bacteria grow mucoid biofilms on the inner surface of the stent (Fig. 14.8). A further complication of this phenomena is halitosis. These stents are also prone to displacement.

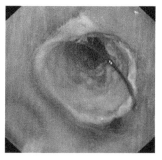

Fig. 14.8a Pseudomonas biofilm formation on a covered endobronchial stent with some mucus plugging.

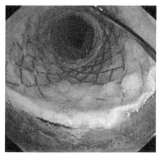

Fig. 14.8b *Early stage of biofilm formation on a covered endobronchial stent.*

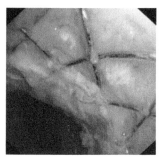

Fig. 14.8c *Close-up view of a covered nitinol stent with early biofilm formation.*

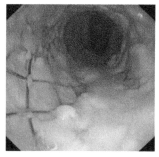

Fig. 14.8d *Development of biofilm with mucus stasis on a covered endobronchial stent.*

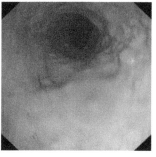

Fig. 14.8e *Progressive development of biofilm with mucus stasis on a covered endobronchial stent.*

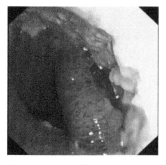

Fig. 14.8f *Granulation tissue developing as a result of an uncovered nitinol stent.*

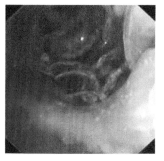

Fig. 14.8g *Granulation tissue at the distal end of an uncovered nitinol stent.*

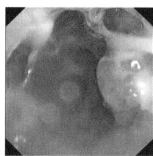

Fig. 14.8h *Granulation tissue developing around an uncovered nitinol stent.*

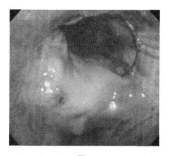

Fig. 14.8i *Tumour growth through an uncovered nitinol stent.*

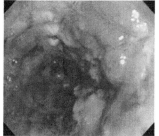

Fig. 14.8j *Tumour ingrowth through an uncovered stent with epithelialization of the stent visible on the other side.*

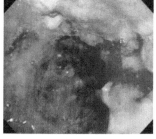

Fig. 14.8k *Tumour recurrence around an epithelialized uncovered stent.*

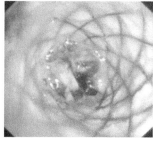

Fig. 14.8l *Distal tumour recurrence in an uncovered stent.*

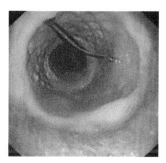

Fig. 14.8m *Covered nitinol stent in the main bronchus, with mucus plugging visible on the inner surface of the stent due to impaired mucociliary clearance.*

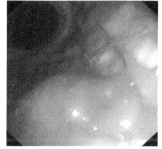

Fig. 14.8n *Mucus collection on a covered stent.*

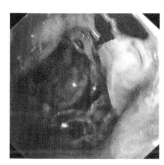

Fig. 14.8o *Stent fracture – a nitinol stent has warped in areas with stent fractures.*

Other complications of stents include development of granulation tissue and overgrowth from the tumour itself at the proximal and distal margins. The stents are exposed to significant forces during coughing and also through the respiratory cycle (Fig. 14.9). Stent fractures are a potential complication and a difficult problem as the stent needs to be removed, usually piecemeal by removing the individual wires carefully with a rigid bronchoscope.

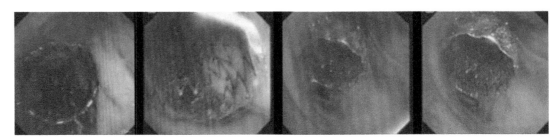

Fig. 14.9a *Migration of stent inserted into the right main bronchus. With coughing the stent moves up into the trachea.*

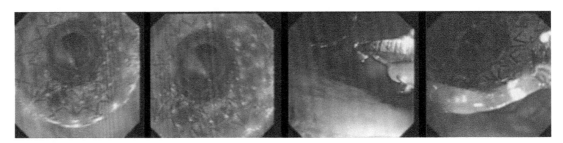

Fig. 14.9b *The stent has migrated to the trachea and is then removed by grasping with biopsy forceps.*

Balloon dilators

In some patients with extrinsic narrowing and also in some patients with circumferential submucosal disease causing airway obstruction, airway dilatation is first required prior to stent insertion. This can be achieved with balloon dilators. Several sizes of balloon dilators are available. Once again I would recommend performing the flexible bronchoscopy in a patient who has been intubated with an uncuffed endotracheal tube.

The balloons are inflated with a pressurized saline-filled syringe. This syringe increases the pressure to a specified amount depending on the degree of dilatation required. The majority of endotracheal balloon dilatations require an interventional bronchoscope with at least a 2.8 mm instrument channel. The balloon is passed through the instrument channel of the bronchoscope and then manipulated through the narrowed airway under direct vision (Fig. 14.10). Once the balloon is appropriately positioned, it is inflated to the set pressure. This should normally be performed in a stepwise dilatation (for example, from 6 to 8 to 10 mm in three separate inflations).

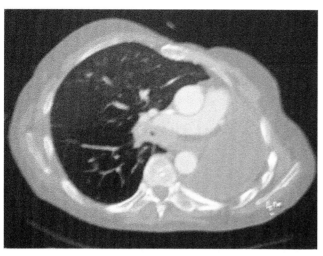

Fig. 14.10a *CT scan in a patient with left pneumonectomy and narrowed right main bronchus.*

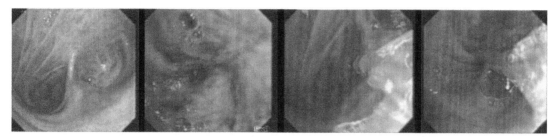

Fig. 14.10b *Circumferential narrowing of the right main bronchus in a patient with left-sided pneumonectomy. Insertion of balloon dilator through the narrowed right main bronchus.*

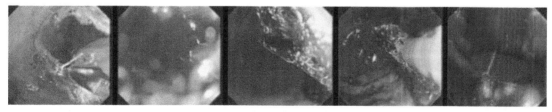

Fig. 14.10c *Inflation of a balloon dilator which has been inserted through the narrowed right main bronchus. There is partial improvement in calibre in the right main bronchus.*

CHAPTER

15

Bronchoscopic treatment for emphysema and asthma: bronchoscopic lung volume reduction

In patients with severe end-stage emphysema, hyperinflation – and particularly dynamic hyperinflation during exertion – is the main cause of dyspnoea and exercise limitation. Patients who are symptomatic despite maximal medical therapy who have undergone pulmonary rehabilitation may be considered for bronchoscopic lung volume reduction. Bronchoscopic techniques and treatment adopted depend on the pattern of emphysema. The majority of patients who have severe emphysema have homogenous disease and about 25 per cent of patients have heterogenous disease.

Heterogenous disease

This is defined as greater than 10 per cent variation in the emphysematous destruction between the upper and lower lobes. A more accurate way of assessing this is by applying a density mask to lung windows and areas with an attenuation value of less than 910 Houndsfield units on 10 mm computed tomography (CT) sections (Fig. 15.1).

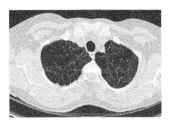

Fig. 15.1a *CT scan showing emphysematous destruction in the upper lobes.*

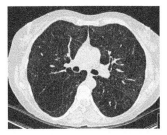

Fig. 15.1b *CT scan from the same patient with emphysema showing relatively less destruction from emphysema.*

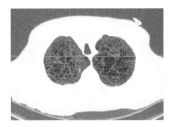

Fig. 15.1c *Density mask highlighting areas with emphysema (> 910 Houndsfield units): in the upper lobe.*

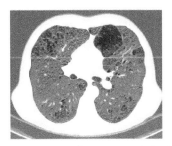

Fig. 15.1d *Density mask highlighting areas with emphysema (> 910 Houndsfield units): in the lower lobe.*

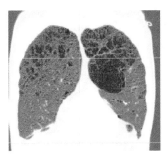

Fig. 15.1e *CT scans showing a greater degree of emphysema in the upper lobes than in the lower lobes: coronal section.*

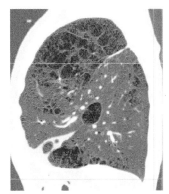

Fig. 15.1f *CT scans showing a greater degree of emphysema in the upper lobes than in the lower lobes: sagittal section.*

● Zephyr valve

The strategy of lobar atelectasis has been utilized with this valve. Hence the recommendation is that the whole of the lobe is treated in a unilateral manner. This is one of the third-generation valves that can be easily inserted through the instrument channel of a bronchoscope. It is available in two main sizes: 4–7 mm and 5.5–8.5 mm.

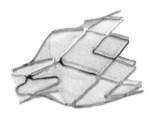

Fig. 15.2a *Zephyr valve.*

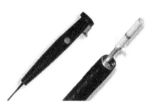

Fig. 15.2b *Delivery catheter handle with a blue button that needs to be pressed prior to pressing the blue lever to slowly deliver the valve. The tip has side blue flanges measuring 4 mm (small flanges) to 7 mm (larger side flanges) which allow you to determine if the valve is the correct size for the target airway segment.*

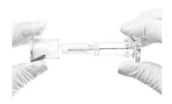

Fig. 15.2c *Valve loading device. The valve is moved into the narrow loading funnel by pulling at the two ends of the device.*

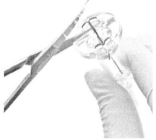

Fig. 15.2d *The retaining thread is cut.*

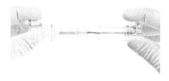

Fig. 15.2e *The funnel with the Zephyr valve in the channel is removed from the capsule.*

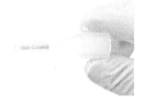

Fig. 15.2f *The Zephyr valve in funnel channel.*

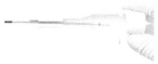

Fig. 15.2g *The delivery catheter positioned in the loading device.*

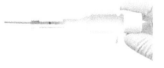

Fig. 15.2h *The delivery catheter positioned in the loading device and pulled down into the narrow channel.*

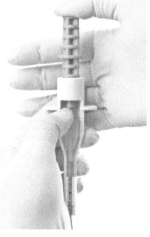

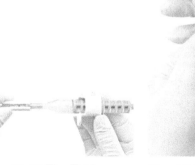

Fig. 15.2i *The Zephyr valve inserted into the loading device.*

Fig. 15.2j *Pusher used to push the valve from the funnel-like capsule into the delivery catheter.*

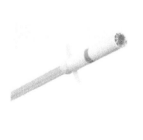

Fig. 15.2k *The Zephyr valve loaded into the distal end of the delivery catheter.*

Sizing is not as critical with Zephyr valves as it is with intrabronchial valves. The delivery catheter has two flanges which provide an estimate of the airway size and therefore the valve that is required. The catheter is placed centrally in the appropriate segment and an estimate can be made using the side flanges to determine which valve should be used.

Once the valve is loaded into the delivery catheter, it is manoeuvred into the appropriate airway segment (Figs 15.2 and 15.3). We recommend using the technique of partial deployment. The valve is very slightly deployed so that it protrudes through the distal tip of the delivery catheter. The valve can then be wedged against the carina within the segment to be treated and deployed. This ensures that the valve is correctly positioned so as to occlude the whole segment. Full deployment in a single manoeuvre can sometimes force the valve into a particular subsegment leading to only partial closure of the segment and this in turn will prevent full lobar atelectasis.

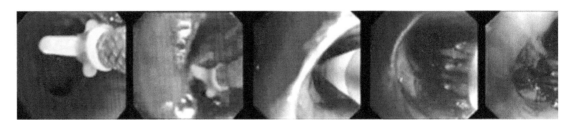

Fig. 15.3a *Delivery catheter for the Zephyr valve with blue side flanges measuring 4 mm (smallest flange) and 7 mm (largest flange). Measurement of the airway segment with a 4 mm catheter demonstrates that the segment diameter is larger than the small flange (4 mm) and smaller than the larger (7 mm) flange and hence suitable for a 4 mm valve, which has a range of 4–7mm. The delivery catheter with a blue margin demarcating the proximal limit of the valve.*

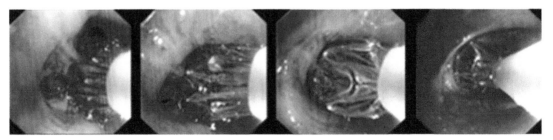

Fig. 15.3b *Slow deployment of the Zephyr valve after wedging against a subsegmental carina.*

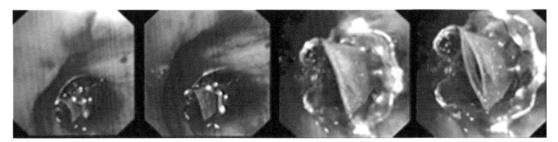

Fig. 15.3c *The Zephyr valve which is closed in inspiration and open in expiration, therefore allowing air out.*

The valves can be easily removed with grasping forceps. The proximal duck-billed valve can be grasped with the forceps and the valve pulled out as a whole unit with the bronchoscope.

The main complications observed are acute exacerbations. Other acute complications include a pneumothorax. In the long term, development of granulation tissue around the valves has been observed. In some cases, there may be secondary colonization of the valves with bacteria such as *Pseudomonas* or fungal species such as *Aspergillus* (Fig. 15.4).

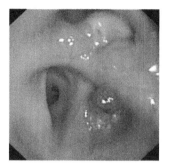

Fig. 15.4a *Granulation tissue around the valve in RB2 and the valve in RB1 has been colonized with Aspergillus.*

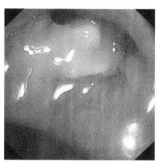

Fig. 15.4b *Close-up of a Zephyr valve colonized with Aspergillus.*

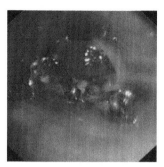

Fig. 15.4c *Another example of granulation tissue developing around the valve.*

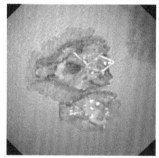

Fig. 15.4d *Zephyr valves covered with a biofilm of mucoid Pseudomonas.*

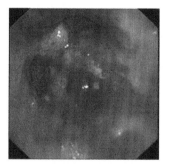

Fig. 15.4e *Appearance of the right upper lobe after removal of Zephyr valves.*

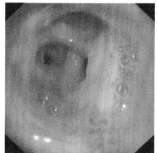

Fig. 15.4f *Appearance of the right upper lobe 6 weeks after removal of Zephyr valves. Note the significant regression of granulation tissue.*

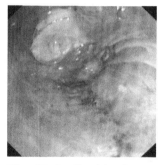

Fig. 15.4g *Combination of granulation tissue and biofilm formation around first-generation duck-billed valve.*

● *Intrabronchial valve*

The intrabronchial valve is an umbrella-shaped device, which is available in sizes of 5, 6 and 7 mm (Fig. 15.5). The manufacturers have been promoting the strategy of airflow re-direction and hence recommend that one subsegment is left patent on the right side and the lingular is untreated on the left side. The valves have a lower margin of error as oversizing causes ruffling of the valve and hence incompetence. Undersizing does not allow a proper seal of the airway either. The valve therefore requires accurate sizing of the airways using a balloon sizing kit.

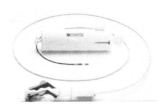

Fig. 15.5a *Loading device and delivery catheter.*

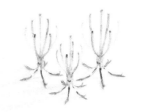

Fig. 15.5b *Intrabronchial valves (5 mm valve in centre, 6 mm valve on left and 7 mm valve on the right side).*

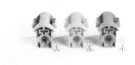

Fig. 15.5c *Intrabronchial valves with colour-coordinated housing: 5 mm valve (blue), 6 mm valve (yellow) and 7 mm valve (green).*

Airway sizing

Balloon preparation and calibration

All the air has to be extracted from the balloon and replaced with normal saline. A three-way tap is attached to the balloon catheter with a 10 mL syringe, which is filled with approximately 5 mL of normal saline. Strong suction is applied so as to remove as much air as possible from the balloons. The balloon is then filled with normal saline (Fig. 15.6). Any air bubbles still present are gently manipulated to the centre of the balloon and suction is applied to the syringe in an attempt to aspirate the gas bubbles. This process is then repeated until there are no air bubbles present or, alternatively, the bubble present in the catheter is smaller than the inner stem of the balloon catheter.

Fig. 15.6a *Balloon catheter.*

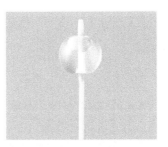

Fig. 15.6b *Balloon catheter inflated with saline but with a significant air bubble.*

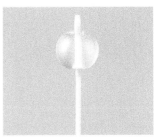

Fig. 15.6c *Balloon catheter with multiple small bubbles (air extracted by repeated suction).*

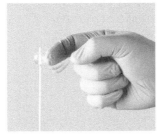

Fig. 15.6d *Gently flicking the balloon encourages the small bubbles to coalesce and form larger bubbles that may be removed by repeated suctioning and inflation of the saline-filled balloon.*

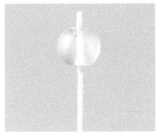

Fig. 15.6e *A single bubble smaller than the diameter of the catheter is acceptable for calibration and sizing.*

The syringe is then exchanged for a 500 µL glass syringe and filled with exactly 500 µL of normal saline. The saline-filled balloon is then calibrated using a sizing template. The balloon is carefully inserted and inflated to fit different-sized templates from 3, 5, 7 and 9 mm holes and the volume of saline in the glass syringe is recorded for each size (Fig. 15.7). In this way a calibration curve for the particular balloon is produced which can then be used to size the airways in a patient.

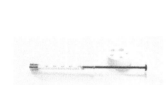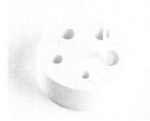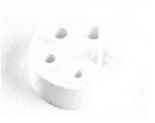

Fig. 15.7a *Calibration template and 500µL glass syringe.*

Fig. 15.7b *The balloon is slowly inflated at each template size. Here, partial inflation of the balloon at the 9 mm hole can be seen.*

Fig. 15.7c *The balloon optimally inflated to 9 mm size template (the volume required to inflate the balloon to this size read from glass syringe).*

Patient preparation

Intubation of all patients undergoing the procedure is recommended. This provides a secure airway but also facilitates removal of valves if required during the procedure. The treatment sites are usually planned according to the findings of a spiral CT scan and a ventilation–perfusion scan. The lobes with the greatest destruction are targeted. The calibration balloon is inserted through the instrument channel and inflated in the target segments until the balloon fits snugly in the segment (Fig. 15.8). The balloon is then moved back and forth in order to determine whether the balloon is correctly inflated. Overinflation leads to some indentation in the balloon. Where there is underinflation a gap may be visible.

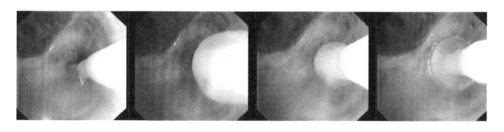

Fig. 15.8a *Balloon catheter inserted into a bronchial segment. Balloon inflated in the bronchial segment and then moved back and forth in the segment. The balloon is optimally inflated to the size of the airway.*

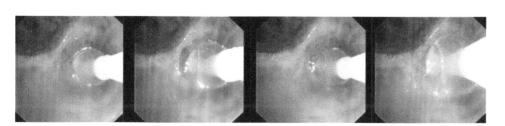

Fig. 15.8b *The optimally inflated balloon moved back and forth in the bronchial segment.*

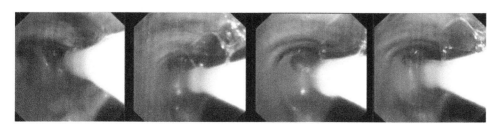

Fig. 15.8c *Note a gap between the segment and the balloon, indicating under-inflation, and then note the slight dimpling in balloon indicating overinflation.*

Procedure

The valve is loaded on to the delivery catheter (Fig. 15.9). This in turn is inserted through the instrument channel of the bronchoscope. Some adjustment of the delivery rod in the trachea is required under direct vision. The catheter is then manoeuvred into the desired segmental airway. The delivery catheter has a proximal marker and is manipulated so that it is appropriately positioned. The valve is delivered and the catheter removed (Fig. 15.10). The valve should be inspected to ensure that it has been correctly placed and that it is fully open with minimal ruffling of the edges of the umbrella. It does tend to retract back by about 1 mm after a few hours. Hence, it is important to check that any side branches or subsegments are fully occluded with an overlap of more than 2 mm. If the valve is oversized then the umbrella tends to be ruffled and not fully open which leads to incompetence of the valve. Similarly if the valve is undersized, the valve tends to leak.

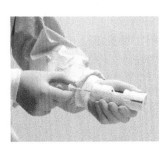

Fig. 15.9a *Plunger retracted in the loading device.*

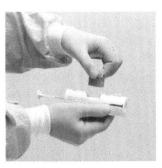

Fig. 15.9b *A 7 mm (green) valve inserted into the loading device.*

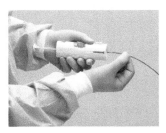

Fig. 15.9c *Delivery catheter inserted into the loading device.*

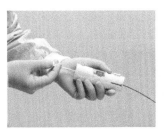

Fig. 15.9d *Plunger pushed into the loading device to transfer the valve into the delivery catheter.*

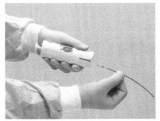

Fig. 15.9e *Delivery catheter released from the loading device by pushing down the yellow button.*

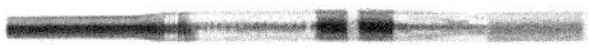

Fig. 15.9f *Intrabronchial valve loaded into the delivery catheter.*

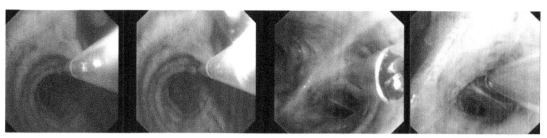

Fig. 15.10a *Delivery catheter inserted into the left main bronchus. There is a small gap between the delivery rod and the valve that is closed in the delivery catheter. The catheter is advanced into the left apicoposterior segment (LB1 + 2) of the upper lobe.*

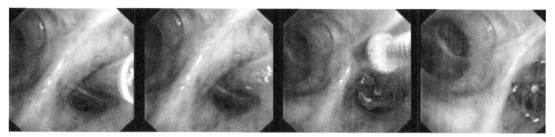

Fig. 15.10b *The delivery catheter is slowly withdrawn back and the yellow line (proximal marker for valve leaflet) is positioned at the origin of the bronchial segment. The valve deployed in left apicoposterior segment (LB1 + 2) of the upper lobe.*

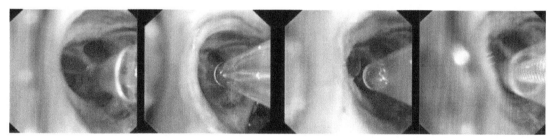

Fig. 15.10c *Catheter tip inserted into the anterior segment of the left upper lobe (LB3).*

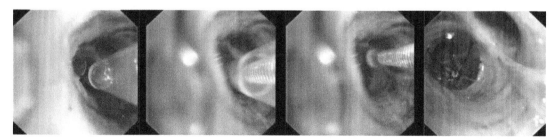

Fig. 15.10d *Valve in the subsegment of the left anterior upper lobe (LB3).*

Valve removal

The intrabronchial valve can be easily removed if it has been incorrectly positioned or if the valve size is incorrect (Fig. 15.11). It can also be removed if the patient does not improve with intervention or if they develop any complications such as post-obstructive infection. The biopsy forceps are inserted through the instrument channel and used to grasp the central rod located on the valve. The valve is then pulled close towards the bronchoscope and the unit is removed in its entirety. Do not attempt to pull the valve through the instrument channel as it will not be possible and there is a risk of damaging the distal portion of the bronchoscope.

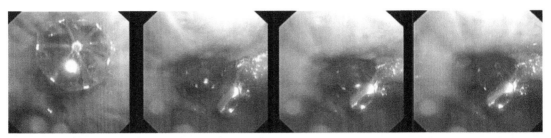

Fig. 15.11a *Incorrectly positioned intrabronchial valve. Removal of valve using biopsy forceps which are first positioned over the intrabronchial valve.*

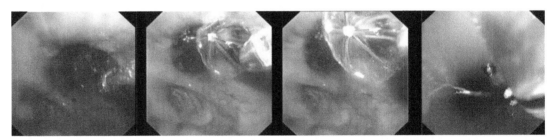

Fig. 15.11b *Biopsy forceps grasp the central rod on the intrabronchial valve. The intrabronchial valve is pulled closer to the bronchoscope and removed through the endotracheal tube as one unit.*

Complications of intrabronchial valve treatment

The most common complication is exacerbation of chronic obstructive pulmonary disease (COPD) which occurs in up to 10 per cent of patients following insertion of endobronchial valves. The patient presents with increased breathlessness, cough, wheezy spells or even mucous hypersecretion. Treatment is with steroids and antibiotics. The other acute complication is that of pneumothorax. It usually resolves with conservative management, requiring intercostal drainage, but only in a small proportion is there a prolonged air leak of more than 7 days. Haemoptysis and haemorrhage are less common and are usually related to incorrect placement of the valve where the protruding section of the valve is rubbing against the airway mucosa. Similarly, valve displacement can occasionally occur but the incidence can be reduced by correct valve replacement. Granulation tissue also develops in some patients with endobronchial valves. We have observed chronic infection such as *Aspergillus* infection around the valve, which usually resolves with removal of the valves.

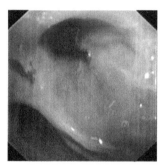

Fig. 15.12a *Granulation tissue enclosing the whole valve with the central rod just visible.*

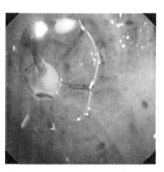

Fig. 15.12b *Mucosal hypertrophy on the lateral aspect of the intrabronchial valve and mucus around the central rod.*

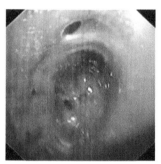

Fig. 15.12c *Almost complete occlusion of the valve by epithelial tissue.*

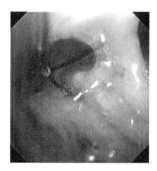

Fig. 15.12d *Mucosal hypertrophy encircling the valve, in particular around the inferior margin.*

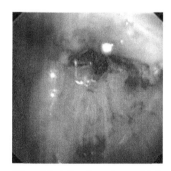

Fig. 15.12e *Intrabronchial valve encircled with tissue hypertrophy.*

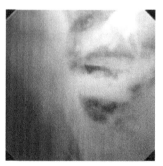

Fig. 15.12f *Colonization of the valve with* Aspergillus.

PneumRx® RePneu® Lung Volume Reduction Coil (LVRC®) System

These are memory coils made from nitinol, which are available in a variety of sizes. Insertion of PneumRx® coils is performed under fluoroscopic guidance during a bronchoscopy (Figs. 15.13 and 15.14).

The coil is a self-actuating device which is delivered straight into the airway. The coil recovers to a non-straight, pre-determined shape upon deployment. The device consists of sterile coils and a sterile, disposable, single-patient delivery system consisting of a cartridge, catheter, guidewire and forceps.

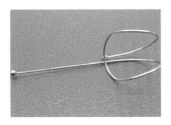

Fig. 15.13a *PneumRx® nitinol coil.*

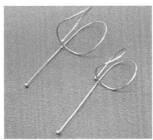

Fig. 15.13b *PneumRx® nitinol coils of differing lengths.*

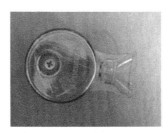

Fig. 15.13c *PneumRx® coil in sterile protective housing.*

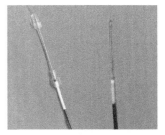

Fig. 15.13d *Catheter and guidewire.*

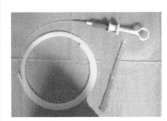

Fig. 15.13e *Grasping forceps with screw (blue) locking mechanism.*

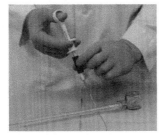

Fig. 15.13f *PneumRx® coil with loading cartridge. Grasped with forceps and locked to prevent inadvertent opening and release of the coil.*

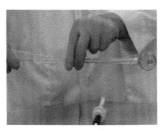

Fig. 15.13g *Coil being loaded into the cartridge by first drawing the grasped coil into the loader.*

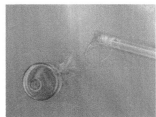

Fig. 15.13h *Coil being loaded into the cartridge.*

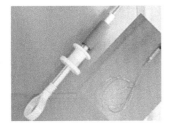

Fig. 15.13i *PneumRx® coil grasped by the forceps. Note the blue screw lock is in the locked position.*

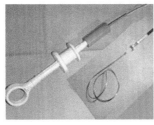

Fig. 15.13j *PneumRx® coil released by the forceps. Note the blue screw lock is in the unlocked position.*

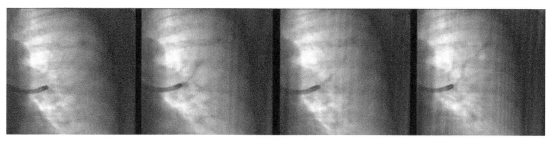

Fig. 15.14a *Catheter inserted into the apicoposterior (LB1 + 2) segment of the left upper lobe. Note the radio-opaque tip of the catheter. PneumRx® coil being advanced through the catheter.*

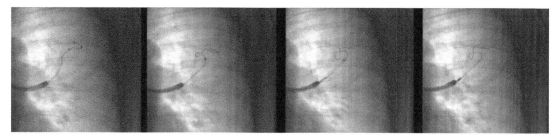

Fig. 15.14b *Overlying catheter being steadily withdrawn with the PneumRx® coil reverting to its original shape. Grasping forceps are visible at the distal end of the bronchoscope.*

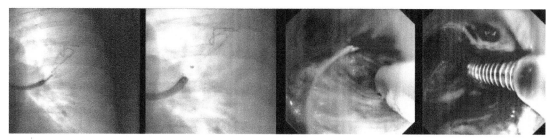

Fig. 15.14c *Grasping forceps are opened releasing the PneumRx® coil. The forceps are then withdrawn. The catheter is repositioned in another airway subsegment and the guidewire is advanced into the bronchial segment.*

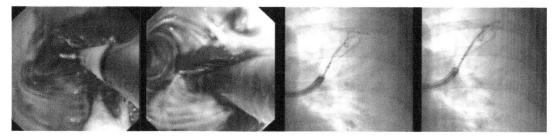

Fig. 15.14d *The guidewire and overlying catheter advanced into the bronchial subsegment.*

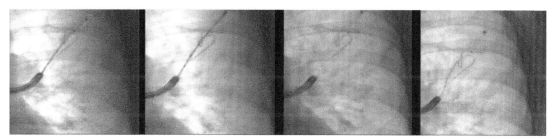

Fig. 15.14e *The catheter being advanced over the guidewire until resistance is felt or the catheter tip is about 3 cm from the pleural edge. The guidewire is withdrawn to the tip of the catheter and the length is estimated with the guidewire which has radio-opaque markers every 25 mm. The guidewire is completely withdrawn leaving the catheter in place.*

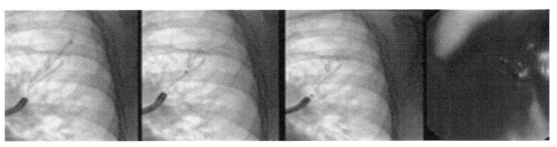

Fig. 15.14f *The PneumRx® coil being advanced through the catheter. The overlying catheter is fully withdrawn with the PneumRx® coil being fully deployed. The distal aspect of the PneumRx® coil is still grasped by forceps.*

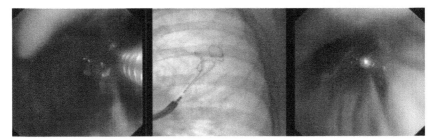

Fig. 15.14g *The grasping forceps are opened to release the PneumRx® coil with the distal tip of PneumRx® coil visible in the airway.*

The procedure can be performed under conscious sedation and ideally the patient should be intubated. The bronchoscope is then passed through the endotracheal tube and manoeuvred towards the target bronchial segment. A catheter with a guidewire is then passed through the instrument channel into the bronchial subsegment. The guidewire is advanced into the bronchial segment under fluoroscopic guidance. The guidewire is inserted until resistance is felt or up to 3 cm from the pleura edge. The catheter is then gently fed over the guidewire to the distal tip of the guidewire. The catheter has a tip that is visible at fluoroscopy and the guidewire has markings every 25 mm along its length that are radiologically visible. The guidewire is then withdrawn back to the tip of the catheter and the distance between the tip of the catheter and the tip of the bronchoscope is calculated from the 25 mm interspaced radiological markers. This allows an estimate of the coil length that should be inserted. The coil is usually oversized by approximately 50 mm.

Adapted bronchial forceps with a locking mechanism are used to grasp the coil and then load it into a specific delivery mechanism and it is fed through the catheter. It is inserted up to the catheter tip under fluoroscopic guidance. The coil is advanced until the distal aspect of the coil reaches the distal point of the catheter and then the overlying catheter is gradually retracted and this allows the coil to conform back to its original shape and in doing so falls and pulls the portion of the lung into which it is inserted. Once the catheter is withdrawn so that the proximal portion of the coil is protruding out of the catheter, the locking mechanism on the biopsy forceps is released and the coil is then released into position. The biopsy forceps can then be removed and the catheter repositioned for the next treatment area. The target lobe is treated systematically with an average of 10 coils.

If a coil is malpositioned then it can be removed or repositioned. The biopsy forceps need to be inserted through the catheter and then used to grasp the small ball-like tip on the proximal aspect of the coil. Once the coil is firmly grasped by its proximal aspect, the biopsy forceps are locked and the catheter is slowly advanced over the coil under fluoroscopic guidance. The re-sheathed coil is effectively straightened and can then be removed or manipulated into a different position.

Ideally a coil should be inserted into each of the subsegments. Hence an upper lobe may be treated with an average of 10 coils.

Homogenous emphysema

In patients with homogenous disease, there is significant destruction of the lung throughout the lung fields. Hence improvements are not based on simply collapsing diseased lung and allowing better lung tissue to function, but more on improvements of chest wall dynamics – in particular, reducing dynamic hyperinflation which is observed on exercise. This group of patients accounts for the majority of patients with severe emphysema.

● Airway bypass

This technique relies on the creation of collateral channels which allow airways of destroyed lung to empty more effectively during expiration and hence reduce hyperinflation. A detailed spiral CT scan is performed first. This allows identification of areas with the most emphysematous lung destruction. Other parameters such as the proximity of blood vessels, airway calibre and bronchoscopic access to the segment are also assessed and scored. A cumulative score is generated to identify the optimal sites of stent insertion.

Procedure

The process is usually performed under general anaesthesia. Airway blockers should be positioned at the start of the procedure to deal with any potential airway haemorrhage. First a Doppler probe is used and positive control is identified by locating an audible Doppler signal or a blood vessel (Figs. 15.15 and 15.16). Then the target area is identified carefully to look for an avascular area (where there is no audible Doppler signal). The bronchoscope is held in position and the Doppler probe removed. A needle with a balloon dilator is then inserted through the bronchoscope channels and inserted into the avascular area identified. The dilator in the needle is inflated and a 3 mm hole is created between the airway segment and the alveolar parenchyma. The balloon is slowly deflated to ensure that there is no significant bleeding. Any minor bleeding is dealt with by gentle suction. If necessary, aliquots of ice-cold saline and diluted adrenaline can be used to control the bleeding.

The area around the newly created passage between the airway and alveolar parenchyma is carefully re-inspected with the Doppler probe to ensure that there are no blood vessels in close proximity to the passage. This is important as release of trapped gas when the hole is made might bring vessels closer than would be safe for stent insertion.

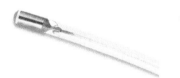

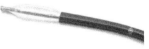

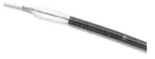

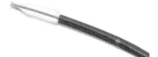

Fig. 15.15a *Exhale® Doppler probe.*

Fig. 15.15b *Exhale® transbronchial dilation needle with the needle withdrawn and the balloon deflated.*

Fig. 15.15c *Exhale® transbronchial dilation needle with the needle protruding and the balloon deflated.*

Fig. 15.15d *Exhale® transbronchial dilation needle with the needle withdrawn and the balloon inflated.*

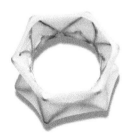

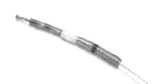

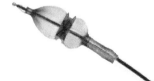

Fig. 15.15e *Exhale® drug-eluting stent.*

Fig. 15.15f *Exhale® drug-eluting stent (white) and underlying balloon mounted on the delivery catheter.*

Fig. 15.15g *Exhale® drug-eluting stent with the inflated balloon delivery catheter.*

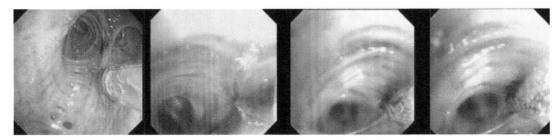

Fig. 15.16a *Exhale® Doppler catheter first identifies a blood vessel (positive control signal to ensure the Doppler probe is functioning). The Exhale® transbronchial dilation needle is inserted through the avascular area identified by the Doppler probe.*

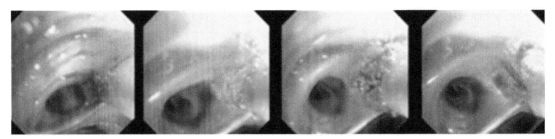

Fig. 15.16b *Balloon dilatation with the Exhale® transbronchial needle after insertion of the needle through the airway into the lung parenchyma.*

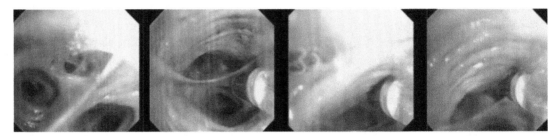

Fig. 15.16c *Hole created by the Exhale® transbronchial needle. The Exhale® Doppler probe checking around the hole created to ensure that it is still free of blood vessels.*

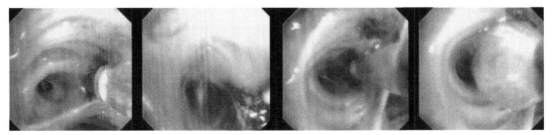

Fig. 15.16d *Exhale® drug-eluting stent on the delivery catheter inserted through the hole created and positioned midway through the stent before balloon inflation. Deployment of the stent by inflation of the balloon catheter. It is important to ensure that black marker on the balloon catheter is visible in order to ensure correct inflation of the balloon.*

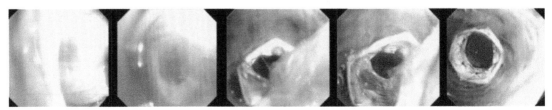

Fig. 15.16e *The stent visible through the dilated balloon. The balloon is deflated after deployment of the stent followed by removal of the delivery catheter. The Exhale® drug-eluting stent supporting the hole that was created. Emphysematous lung is visible through the stent.*

A drug-eluting stent on a balloon catheter is then inserted through the airway passage (Fig. 15.16d). The stent on the delivery catheter is then carefully positioned so that the mid-portion of the stent is just through the bronchial wall. Care should also be taken to ensure the balloon dilator is fully extended out from the distal tip of the bronchoscope and the black marker line on the catheter is visible. Once appropriately positioned, the balloon is inflated to a specific pressure and held in position for at least 10 seconds. The dilation of the balloon deploys the stent and maintains the passage created. The balloon is then slowly deflated and the catheter carefully removed.

The stent should be inspected to ensure that it is correctly positioned and there is no overlying lip of mucosa. The procedure is repeated to create further airway passages and three stents are usually inserted into each lung, with a maximum of two in each lobe.

The procedure is likely to evolve so that in future a combination of a needle dilator and ultrasound transducer will reduce its duration. It is also possible that only two optimally placed stents may be required for clinical benefit.

Occasionally the bronchial tissue may be very friable and this will lead to airway tearing during balloon dilatation. This results in larger holes than are suitable for the airway stent. In such cases, it may be possible to omit the balloon dilatation with the needle and proceed straight to stent deployment. In some cases, the stent may be angulated or not properly deployed and require retrieval. This can be achieved easily with biopsy forceps. We recommend simply passing the biopsy forceps through the displaced channel and then opening the forceps so that the stent is now trapped within them, and removing the bronchoscope, forceps and stent as a single unit.

The main limitation of the stents is that they become occluded over time (usually within 3 months). Figure 15.17 shows epithelialization of the stents in various stages.

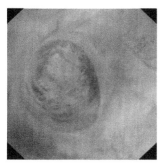

Fig. 15.17a *The stent deployed so that lateral leaflets are embedded in the airway mucosa.*

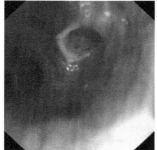

Fig. 15.17b *Epithelium growing over the majority of the stent but still patent.*

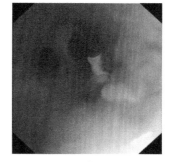

Fig. 15.17c *The stent almost completely embedded within the airway. It was originally deployed in a position where part of the stent was covered with epithelium.*

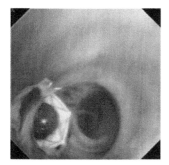

Fig. 15.17d *Membrane completely covering and occluding the stent.*

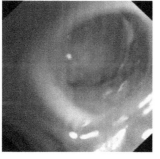

Fig. 15.17e *Membrane covering and occluding the inner surface of the stent.*

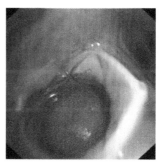

Fig. 15.17f *Combination of epithelium growing over the stent and membrane covering the inner surface.*

Complications

Airway haemorrhage is the most serious potential complication, hence care and attention are required throughout the procedure. It is essential that the Doppler assessment of blood vessels is performed carefully. Any bleeding should be handled as described in the bleeding protocol (Box 12.1, p. 212). In addition, any bleeding noticed during the balloon deflation can be rapidly managed by re-inflating the balloon. The tamponade effect of the balloon should manage and contain the airway bleeding. After the procedure the most common complication observed is exacerbation of COPD or acute bronchitis. Pneumomediastinum is also frequently seen with this procedure, but it is usually self-limiting and does not require any intervention. Pneumothorax is also observed and again this is self-limiting and is usually managed with intercostal drainage.

Bronchial thermoplasty for asthma

Bronchial thermoplasty is a technique that reduces airway smooth muscle in patients with asthma. Treatment reduces the frequency of hospitalization, exacerbations and health care utilization.

The technique uses the Alair radiofrequency controller and Alair catheter, which delivers the energy to the airways (Fig. 15.18). The energy delivered heats up the local tissue to around 65°C and selectively reduces the airway smooth muscle bulk. There is some mucosal oedema which recovers over the next 7–14 days.

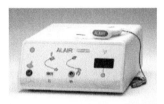

Fig. 15.18a *Alair radiofrequency controller with Alair bronchial thermoplastic catheter.*

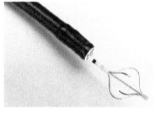

Fig. 15.18b *Distal aspect of the Alair catheter. Note the small bare (not insulated) mid-section of the open catheter.*

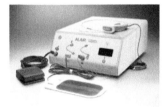

Fig. 15.18c *Alair radiofrequency controller with foot pedal, earthing plate and Alair bronchial thermoplastic catheter.*

The patient has an earthing plate attached to the thigh or lower back. The Alair catheter is introduced through the instrument channel of the bronchoscope and inserted into the most distal accessible airway. Success of the treatment depends on comprehensive treatment of the airway, with care taken not to apply repeated treatments to the same airway. This relies on a systematic approach. In the clinical trials the treatments were administered over three sessions, treating the right lower lobe, the left lower lobe and then the two upper lobes and lingula by bronchoscopy every 3 weeks. Our approach, for example, for the right lower lobe is to treat RB10 (right posterior basal bronchus) first, using the BF260 bronchoscope (external diameter 4.3 mm) so that the distal subsegments can be assessed.

The Alair catheter is passed through the instrument channel and then opened in the distal airway (Fig. 15.19). Once fully in contact with the airway, the foot pedal is activated to deliver the radiofrequency energy in a specific algorithm. The treatment takes about 10 seconds and an audible signal indicates duration and completion of treatment. The wire basket is then partially closed and the catheter moved proximally by about 4 mm and then reopened. This manoeuvre is repeated so that all the airways from the distal aspect to the proximal portion are treated in a stepwise manner. Any side branches that are visualized should also be treated at the same time.

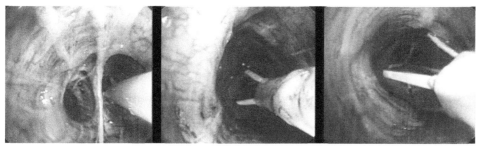

Fig. 15.19a *Alair catheter opened in the distal aspect of the airway. The energy is delivered when the catheter is expanded and in full contact with the airways. The catheter is partially closed and moved proximally by about 4 mm. The catheter is then re-expanded and a further cycle of energy is delivered. In this stepwise manner, the whole length of the airway and any side branches are treated.*

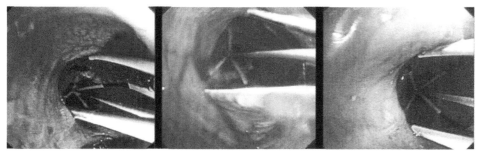

Fig. 15.19b *Alair catheter in contact with the airways. The bare section through which the energy is delivered can be seen. The catheter is fully expanded against the airways. Note the central green wire and four equally spaced, partially insulated wires.*

The radiofrequency controller delivers the energy over a 10-second period and any loss of contact of the catheter from the airway wall, due to coughing etc., will cause the radiofrequency controller to cut out with incomplete delivery of the energy. A further cycle can be delivered at the same site, but if there are two incomplete activations at one individual site then the catheter should be moved more proximally before further treatment.

Patient management is an important step during the bronchoscopy to ensure adequate application of lidocaine through the airways and appropriate sedation to minimize patient movement and coughing.

Once the full segment has been treated, the bronchoscope is systematically moved to the next segment, in this case RB9 (lateral segment of the right lower lobe) then RB8, RB7 and RB6 in sequence. The main adverse events and complications are an exacerbation of the asthma, increased mucous secretions and some mucosal oedema. Mucous plugging and atelectasis are occasionally observed.

Inversion of the wire basket portion of the catheter occasionally occurs and the radiofrequency generator would prevent activation (Fig. 15.20). The wire basket should be visualized at all times and care taken to ensure that it is correctly opened and apposed to the airway wall before the radiofrequency generator is activated to deploy the energy.

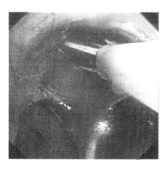

Fig. 15.20a *Inversion of an Alair catheter in the apical segment of the right upper lobe.*

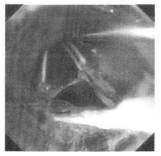

Fig. 15.20b *Close-up of the inverted catheter. Note the green wire is in the superior position and partially insulated wires are inverted and inferior to the green wire.*

Index

Notes

As the subject of this book is bronchoscopy, entries under this term have been kept to a minimum. Readers are advised to look for more definite terms.

Entries for right- or left-sided anatomical structures can be found under right or left, not under the anatomical structure.

To save space in the index, the following abbreviations have been used:

CT – computed tomography; TBNA – transbronchial fine-needle aspiration

basal segments, 64
   electromagnetic navigation, 179, 182
   left lower lobe, 47, 51, 72, 76
   right lower lobe, 43, 44, 64, 66, 68
basement membrane elastin, confocal microscopy, 168
basolateral segments, right lower lobe, 43, 44
bio-fouling, stents, 216, 217
biopsy forceps, 8
   sterilization, 3–4
bipartite division, upper lobe, 37, 38, 56, 62
bleeding see haemorrhage
bleeding diathesis, 5
blood, autofluorescence bronchoscopy, 165
blood vessels
   confocal microscopy, 168
   see also specific vessels
brachiocephalic veins, 78
   endobronchial ultrasound bronchoscopy, 141
brachytherapy, tumour debulking, 209–10
bronchial biopsies, 8
bronchial brushings, 9
bronchial gland, confocal microscopy, 168
bronchial thermoplasty, asthma, 236–7
bronchial tree, CT correlation, 23
bronchial washings, 8
bronchioalveolar cell carcinoma, confocal microscopy, 169
bronchioles, confocal microscopy, 168
bronchoalveolar lavage, 9–10
bronchocentric granulomatosis, 163
bronchopulmonary segments, 11–27
   nomenclature, 11–13
bronchoscopes, 1–2
   diameter, 2, 3
   instrument channels, 2
   linear array ultrasound probes, 2, 3
bronchoscopic lung volume reduction see lung volume reduction
bronchus
   left main see left main bronchus
   lingular see lingular bronchus
   right main see right main bronchus
bronchus intermedius, 39, 60, 63–4
   CT, 24, 39, 42, 61, 64

C

candidiasis, 158
carcinoma in situ, right lower lobe, autofluorescence bronchoscopy, 166
carina, 31, 33–4, 56, 57–8
   CT, 33, 58, 59
   dysplasia, autofluorescence bronchoscopy, 166
   electromagnetic navigation, 173
   left main see left main carina
   main see main carina
   nomenclature, 12
   renal cell carcinoma, 160
   thickening, autofluorescence bronchoscopy, 165
   tracheobronchial amyloid, 160
   tumours, 160

cartilage nodules
   right lower lobe, autofluorescence bronchoscopy, 165
   trachea, 159
cartilage rings, 31
cartilages see specific cartilages
CCDs (charge-coupled devices), 1
cellular composition, bronchoalveolar lavage, 10
charge-coupled devices (CCDs), 1
chronic obstructive pulmonary disease (COPD)
   confocal microscopy, 170
   intrabronchial valve complications, 229
coagulation probe, electrocautery, 202, 203
Cohen endobronchial balloon blocker, 192–3, 192–7
   difficulties, 196–7
   left main bronchus insertion, 194–5, 194–7
colorectal carcinoma, metastases see metastatic colorectal carcinoma
computed tomography (CT)
   anterior TBNA, 94, 95, 96
   balloon dilators, 219
   bronchopulmonary segments, 23–7
   emphysema, 220
   patient preparation, 5
   pre-electromagnetic navigation, 172, 173
   pre-endobronchial ultrasound bronchoscopy, 134
   pre-intrabronchial valve, 225
   pre-TBNA, 113, 114–15
   stent insertion, 212, 213, 215
   see also specific anatomical features
concentric segmental tumour, 161
confocal microscopy, 167–71
   equipment, 167
conscious sedation, PneumRx® coils, 232
consent, 5
contraindications (for bronchoscopy), 5
COPD see chronic obstructive pulmonary disease (COPD)
corniculate cartilage, intubation problems, 191
corniculate tubercle, 30, 55
   CT, 53
   right see right corniculate tubercle
cough technique
   anterior TBNA, 98
   transbronchial fine needle aspiration (TBNA), posterior approach, 117
cricoid cartilage, CT, 53
cross-infection, 3
cryoextraction, 207, 208
cryotherapy, 202, 206–8, 207
CT see computed tomography (CT)
cuneiform cartilage, 28, 53
cuneiform tubercle, 30, 55
   CT, 53
   right see right cuneiform tubercle
cytology
   anterior TBNA, 98
   endobronchial ultrasound bronchoscopy, 156, 157
   TBNA, 98

D

density mask, emphysema, 220
descending aorta, CT, 58, 59
diameter, bronchoscopes, 2, 3
diathermy see electrocautery
diffuse infiltrative carcinoma, 161
diffuse lung disease, 4(Box)
   bronchoalveolar lavage, 9
direct vision, stent insertion, 211–15, 212–15
disinfection, 3–4
disposable instruments, 4
distortion, trachea, 159
drug-eluting stents, airway bypass, 235
drug-related hypersensitivity pneumonitis, confocal microscopy, 170
dysplasia, carina, autofluorescence bronchoscopy, 166

E

elastin network, confocal microscopy, 168
electrocautery, 202–5
   coagulation probe, 202, 203
   complications, 205(Box)
   electrosurgical knife, 202
   electrosurgical snare, 202, 204
   equipment, 202
   hot biopsy forceps, 202, 205
   precautions, 205(Box)
   see also argon plasma coagulation
electromagnetic navigation, 172–88
   advances, 187–8
   equipment, 172
   navigation, 184–6, 184–8
   planning stage, 172–9
   registration process, 180–3
electrosurgical knife, 202
electrosurgical snare, 202, 204
emphysema, 220–37
   confocal microscopy, 169, 170
   CT, 220
   density mask, 220
   heterogenous disease, 220–32
   homogenous, 233–6
   see also airway bypass
endobronchial tumour debulking see tumour debulking
endobronchial tumours
   confocal microscopy, 169
   stents, 216, 217
endobronchial ultrasound bronchoscopy, 133–57
   equipment, 133
   examination approach, 134–5
   hilar zone lymph nodes, 149–53
      left hilar lymph node (Station 11L), 153
      left main bronchial lymph node (Station 10R), 150
      right inferior hilar lymph node (Station 11Ri), 152
      right main bronchial lymph node (Station 10R), 149
      right superior hilar lymph node (Station 11Rs), 151
   inferior mediastinal lymph nodes, 148

Printed and bound by CPI Group (UK) Ltd, Croydon, CR0 4YY

17/10/2024

01775663-0013